PAIN CONTROL

WITH

TRANSCUTANEOUS ELECTRICAL NEURO STIMULATION

PAIN CONTROL
with
TRANSCUTANEOUS ELECTRICAL NEURO STIMULATION (T.E.N.S.)

By

ROBERT A. ERSEK, M.D.(Ed.)
Plastic and Reconstructive Surgery
Bailey Surgical Center
Austin, Texas
Clinical Instructor
University of Texas
Medical Branch at San Antonio
Division of Plastic and Reconstructive Surgery

WARREN H. GREEN, INC.
St. Louis, Missouri, U.S.A.

Published by

WARREN H. GREEN, INC.
8356 Olive Blvd.
St. Louis, Missouri 63132, U.S.A.

Library of Congress Catalog Card No. 78-50175
ISBN No. 0-87527-168-5

Printed in the United States of America

To my wife Gerry and daughters
Stephanie and Cynthia
and
To our patients
from whom we learn.

CONTRIBUTORS

Gail H. Baumgartner, A.B.
Medical Writer - Editor
New Orleans, Louisiana

Alan V. Bornstein, Ph. D.
Pain Clinic
Jersey Shore Medical Center
West Deal, New Jersey

Joseph G. Bussey, M.D., F.A.C.S.
Assistant Clinical Professor of Surgery
Director, Pain and Rehabilitation Center
Emory University
Douglasville, Georgia

Ross Davis, M.D.
Chief of Neurological Surgery
Mount Sinai Medical Center
and Variety Childress Hospital
Miami Beach, Florida

Melvin Denholtz, D.D.S.
Chief, Dental Research
Newark Beth Israel Hospital
Newark, New Jersey

Robert A. Ersek, M.D.
Plastic and Reconstructive Surgery
Bailey Surgical Center
Austin, Texas

Alan C. Hymes, M.D.
Cardiovascular and Thoracic Surgery
Methodist and Mount Sinai Hospitals
Minneapolis, Minnesota

Walter Indeck, M.D.
Department of Orthopeadic Surgery
St. Louis Park Medical Center &
University of Minnesota Medical School
Minneapolis, Minnesota

Amy Jackson, R.N., P.A.
Emory University
Douglasville, Georgia

Estelle Kornhauser, R.N.
Staff Nurse
Pain Control Center
Silver Springs, Maryland

Roman Kurzbauer, M.D.
Head, Surgical Department
Prudnik County Hospital
Prudnik, Poland

Gerald N. Lampe, R.P.T., B.S.
Instructor, Penn Valley Community College
Kansas City, Missouri

Richard Lentini, M.S.
Research Associate
Miami Beach, Florida

John Miles, M.B., B. Ch., F.R.C.S.
University of Liverpool
Consultant Neurosurgeon
Regional Department of Medical and Surgical Neurology
Walton Hospital
Liverpool, England

Boleslaw Rutkowski, M.D.
Head, Department of Anestesiology
Oncological Institute in Gliwice
Head, Pain Relief Clinic
Integrated Health Care Complex
Gliwice, Poland

Gerald D. Schuster, M.D.
Clinical Assistant Professor Orthopaedic Surgery
Georgetown University Medical School
Consulting Physician in Orthopaedic Surgery
Veterans Administration Hospital
Washington, D.C.

C. Norman Shealy, M.D., Ph.D.
Director, Pain and Health Rehabilitation Center
Clinical Associate
Department of Psychology
University of Wisconsin,
LaCrosse, Wisconsin

Gary D. VanderArk, M.D.
Clinical Assistant Professor
Department of Surgery
University of Colorado Medical Center
Denver, Colorado

INTRODUCTION

ALAN C. HYMES, M.D.

The thing that hath been, it is that which shall be; and that which is done is that which shall be done: And there is no new thing under the sun.
Ecclesiastes 1, 9

Over the past decade, there has been a resurgence of electrotherapy in various forms. But, this is not a new theory or technique. Since the discovery of electricity. . . . and indeed, from the time of Hippocrates and Scribonius Largus' utilization of the torpedo fish therapeutically in 46 A.D. (1,2) the interest has grown.

William Gilbert, 1544 to 1603 first classified and generalized the phenomenon of electricity (3). From that time, a multitude of apparatuses were made to generate and store current, which was applied, in various forms, to all parts of the body for a multiplicity of afflictions (3,4).

Richard Lovett published the *Subtil Medium Proved* in 1756 (3). It was the first English language book on medical electricity in which he listed dozens of cures for many diseases.

But the man who primarily influenced this Introduction is John Wesley, religious leader, and founder of the Methodist Church. He became extremely enthusiastic with this mode of medical treatment. Personally a clinician and investigator in electrotherapy, in 1759 he published his Desideratum: or *Electricity made plain and useful by a lover of mankind and of common sense* (5). Wesley saw the "subtle fluid" as the soul of the universe, giving many examples of diseases which were "cured" by the use of electrotherapy. Included among the ailments were sciatica, hysteria, headache, kidney stone, gout, cold feet (Raynaud's phenomenon), pleuritic pain, and angina pectoris.

He (2) ended the *Desideratum* with the following plea which seems to me most fitting in this introduction:

> *"Before I conclude, I would beg one Thing (If it be not too great a Favour) from the Gentlemen of the Faculty, and indeed from all who desire Health and Freedom from Pain, either for themselves, or their Neighbors. It is, That none of them would condemn they know not what: That they would hear the Cause, before they pass Sentence: That they would not preemptorily pronounce against Electricity, while they know little or nothing about it. Rather let every candid Man take a little Pains, to understand the Question before he*

determines it. Let him for two or three weeks (at least) try it himself in the above named Disorders. And then his own Senses will show him, whether it is a mere Play-thing, or the noblest Medicine yet known in the World."

As quoted from Calaway (3) between the years 1750 and 1780 there were 26 publications dealing with clinical electricity. A new electrical shock machine was installed in the Middlesex Hospital in 1767.

Mr. John Birch (6), an English surgeon, in 1772 described the methods by which he applied electrical current and gave case histories. He utilized current for a hand injury on an 18 year old boy in pain and contractions. After a few sessions, the boy regained full function of the hand and the pain disappeared. There were a number of examples cited of treatment of chronic low back pain and "perfect" cures. He also detailed the treatment of chronic constipation by placing a young female patient in an electrical chair. Her second treatment resulted in an evacuation of bowels in five minutes with the application of current. There were also successful case histories relative to treatment of gout and other afflictions.

In 1875, the second edition of Rockwell, Byrd, and Rockwell was published (7). In this book, they summarized the history of electrotherapy. Included is a long description directing their application of treatment and reminding them of their responsibility in the utilization of electrotherapy. There are multiple chapters of specifics relative to system-related diseases. These included asthmatic diseases, rheumatism, gout, progressive muscular dystrophy, local motor ataxia, neuralgia, migraine, and pain back. Also included were such afflictions as alcoholism and many gastrointestinal tract disorders, and skin diseases. Included was a specific chapter on neuralgia, consisting chiefly of case reports and treatment of low back pain by electrical stimulation. Scars and ulcerations of the skin were noted to be complications in chronic conditions.

It is interesting to note that electrotherapy had little use in the mainstream of modern medicine in the past 70 years, in spite of the well documented use of this modality in previous times. As such, little clinical research and no publications have appeared in medical literature until very recently.

Basic research,however, was being conducted by numerous

investigators during this time as reviewed by Pfeiffer (8).

Licht (9) reviewed the available historical literature and reported this comprehensive study in 1967 citing over 900 references.

Since the early 1900's, apparatuses such as "Electreat" were sold directly to consumers by the manufacturer without physician evaluation. These instruments also became popular among chiropractors and other practitioners of medicine who were held in poor esteem. All types of curative claims were ascribed to these units including the cure of cancer. Subsequently, the FDA banned their sale in the early 1950's.

Neurophysiological research (10,11,12,13,14) in the late 50's and early 60's led to the Gate Theory of pain as proposed by Melzack and Wall (15).

Basically, the Gate Theory states that nonpainful stimulation in the peripheral nervous system can interfere with the relay of the sensation of pain to higher centers. This block occurs within the central nervous system. Thus, the theory may explain in part why peripheral electrical stimulation may diminish or abolish the sensation of pain.

Shealy reasoned that direct stimulation of the dorsal column of the spinal cord could inhibit the spread of pain impulses to higher perception areas. He experimented with cats and monkeys and found that the pain threshold was increased significantly (13). Subsequently, Shealy *et al.* reported the first clinical use of a dorsal column implantation (16). It was described in a patient with recurrent metastatic carcinoma of the lung, who had intractable pain. Since then, neurosurgeons throughout the world have implanted dorsal column and anterior column electrodes for stimulation. Recently, Burton (17) has implanted electrodes percutaneously in the dorsal columns of the spinal cord.

Initially, it was difficult to predict which patients would respond favorably to dorsal column stimulation. Don Long (18,19) and C. N. Shealy (5,20) in collaboration and independently have developed means for evaluating patients for dorsal column implantation by Transcutaneous Electrical Neuro Stimulation (TENS). Many patients, noting that TENS seemed to reduce the perception of pain prefer it to the dorsal column implant. As such, many patients have been treated successfully with this modality. It became an important part of the Pain Clinic which Long established at the University of Minnesota, and now at Johns Hopkins University, and Shealy's Clinic in LaCrosse, Wisconsin.

At this point, private industry entered with a tremendous amount of vital participation in the growth and development of TENS. Many companies were involved. We in the field owe them a debt of gratitude for their support, making various clinical studies possible throughout the country, and developing instrumentation which became an integral part of our investigations.

The concept of the utilization of electricity to alleviate pain has been with us for centuries. It has simply taken divergent paths which have led us to today's perspective.

T.E.N.S. can serve as a non-invasive, non-pharmacologic means whereby man's pain may be controlled, which may ultimately lead him to the capability of finding the inner resources to bring him in touch with his reality of being.

In the end, every individual is responsible for himself, and has the capacity within himself to find reasonable means of alleviating his own suffering, no matter what its source, if he so chooses. T.E.N.S. is one such modality. The choice is man's.

BIBLIOGRAPHY

1. *Hagbarth, K.E. Kerr. D.:* Central Influences on Spinal Afferent Conduction. *J. Neurophysiol., 17*:295, 1954
2. Schonoch, W.:*Die rezept Sammlung des Scribonius.* Jena, 1912-13
3. Stillings, D.: *A Short History of Electrotherapy in England to about 1880.* 1974. Museum of Electricity in Life at Medtronic.
4. Stillings, D.: A survey of the History of Electrical Stimulation for Pain to 1900. *Medical Instrum., 9*:255, 1975
5. Shealy, C.M.: Six Years' Experience with Electrical Stimulation for Control of Pain. *Adv. In Neuro., 4:*755, 1974.
6. Birch, J.: *Essay on Electricity. . . .*by George Adams. 4th Ed. p. 519, 1772. Pub. R. Hindmarsh, London. Museum of Electricity in Life at Medtronic
7. Rockwell, Burton, Byrd, G.M. and Rockwell, A.D.: *A Practical Treatise on the Medical and Surgical Uses of Electricity.* 2nd Ed. 1975, Wm. Wood & Co. Pub.
8. Pfeiffer, E.: Electric Stimulation of Sensory Nerves with Skin Electrodes for Research, Diagnosis, Communication and Behavorial Conditioning: *A Survey. Med. & Biol. Engng., 6:*637, 1968.
9. Licht, S.: Therapeutic Electricity and Ultraviolet Irradiation. *History of Electrotherapy. Physical Med. Library., 4*:1, 1967. Pub. Elisabeth Licht, New Haven, Conn.

10. Collins, W.F., Randt, C.T.: Evoked Central Nervous System Activity Relating to Peripheral Unmyelinated or "C" Fibers in the Cat. *J. Neurophysiol.*, *21*:345, 1958.
11. Sweet, W.H., Wepsic, J.G.: Treatment of Chronic Pain by Stimulation of Fibers of Primary Afferent Neuron. *Trans. Amer. Neurol. Assn.*, *93*:103, 1968.
12. Poggio, G.F., Mountcastle, V.B.: A Study of the Functional Contributions of the Lemniscal and Spinothalmic Systems to Somatic Sensibility. *Bull.Johns Hopkins Hosp.*, *106:*266, 1960.
13. Shealy, C.N.: The Physiological Substrate of Pain. *Headache*,*6*:101, 1966.
14. Wall, P.D.: The Laminar Organization of Dorsal Horn and Effects of Descending Impulses. *J. Physiol.* (London), *188*:403, 1967.
15. Melzack, R., Wall: Pain Mechanisms; A New Theory. *Science*, *150*:971, 1965.
16. Shealy, C.N., Mortimer, J.T., Reswich, J.B.: Electrical Inhibition of Pain by Stimulation of the Dorsal Column: Preliminary Clinical Reports. *Anesth. Analg.*, *45*:489, 1967.
17. Burton, C.: Percutaneous Radiofrequency. Facet Denervation. *J. Applied Neurophysiol.* In press.
18. Long, D.M.: Recent Advances in the Management of Pain. *Minn. Med.*, *56*:705, 1974.
19. Long, D.M.: External Electrical Stimulation as a Treatment of Chronic Pain. *Minn. Med.*, *57*:195, 1974.
20. Shealy, C.N.: Transcutaneous Electroanalgesia. *Surg. For.*, *23*:419, 1973.

ACKNOWLEDGMENTS

A note of appreciation to Mr. Dennis Stillings, Director of the Museum of Electricity in Life at Medtronic, and especially to Mr. Earl Bakken whose imagination and generosity made the museum possible.

CONTENTS

PAIN CONTROL

WITH

TRANSCUTANEOUS ELECTRICAL NEURO STIMULATION

Chapter 1

THE HISTORY AND DEVELOPMENT OF ELECTROANALGESIA

ROBERT A. ERSEK, M.D., and GAIL H. BAUMGARTNER, A.B.

Transcutaneous Electrical Neuro Stimulation, the basis for this series of discussions, will be examined as to its evolution, areas of usage, and efficacy as a non-toxic, non-pharmacologic therapy for the relief of a number of acute and chronic pain states.

Its roots lie in the basic concepts of electro-analgesia. Today we are striving to overcome the communication problem which stems from the lack of a standard terminology for pain syndromes, and the absence of adequate national and international pain data pools. That would facilitate evaluation and discussion of past and present forms of therapy. However, hope lies in the fact that basic scientists as well as clinicians involved in teaching, research, and patient care have joined together to create multidisciplinary pain groups (1).

The "shocking" concept - electricity - had its beginning in Socratic times. Scribonius Largus claimed to cure arthritis and headaches with the application of electric-torpedo fish in the first century. The therapeutic belief in electro-analgesia continued throughout the Middle Ages. Avicenna and Averrhoes advocated its utilization for arthralgia and cephalgia. Dawd al Antaki (16th century) even in dire situations used the torpedo fish in the treatment of chronic headache, vertigo, and unilateral headache. When electricity was controllable by Otto von Guericke's electrostatic sulphur sphere, Haukshbee invented an electrostatic generator. This was used in combination with the Leyden jar condensors of von Kleist and van Musschenbroek (1745-46).

Electricity's application for the treatment of pain continued through the ages. There was great development in the

18th century. Reverend John Wesley treated such complaints as gout, headaches, and sciatica by applying electricity using the electrostatic generator and Leyden jar. The concept of electro-stimulation was in the minds of Wesley and his colleagues, and we find frequent records of electrical means of treatment. These men had evolved the idea that the electric fire dilated the minute vessels and capillary passages, as well as separating the clogged particles of the stagnating fluids. By "electrification," the motion of the blood was thought to be accelerated and many obstructions were removed.

Oriental acupuncture became known to the Western world, and Sarlandiere published his work on the mechanisms of pain relief by electroacupuncture in the 19th century (2).

The use of electroshock therapy as a modality of treatment for psychiatric depression is a profound form of pain modulation by electro-stimulation.

The concept of therapeutic usages of electricity continues to expand. Dr. Hymes, in his Introduction, cites other references.

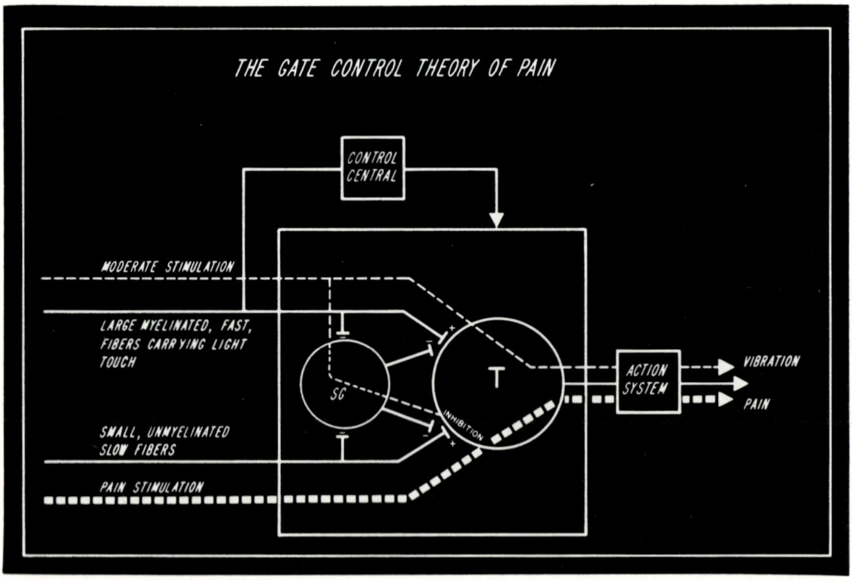

Figure 1. Gate Control Theory

With the proposal of the Gate Control Theory by Melzack and Wall in 1965, a rational basis for electro-analgesia was postulated. They produced evidence which showed the dull, slow, diffuse, burning pain is carried from the periphery by small, primative, unmyelinated fibers, while the sensation of light touch is carried by large myelinated fibers. The sensory output carried along these two sets of fibers from a given location were modulated in the substantia gelatinosa of the dorsal horns within the spinal cord and acted upon each other as a negative feedback mechanism (3) (Figure 1). By forcing the large A fibers to carry light touch sensation by electrical stimulation of the area, pain signals from the C fibers were blocked even after the electrical stimulation stopped.

At Harvard, in 1967, Wall and Sweet (4) applied the Gate Control theory clinically using implanted stimulating devices through low voltage, percutaneous electrical stimulation of themselves. This work then led to stimulation of the peripheral nerves or the posterior cord for pain control (5,6).

It became apparent that not all pain patients were suited for implantation or the accompanying risks of any surgical procedure, The pain persisted. In an endeavor to discover a test for the ultimate success or failure of implantable devices for stimulation, work was begun investigating transcutaneous applications of electrical stimulation for pain relief. As a result of the early successes of the crude, commercially available stimulators, concentrated effort was made toward the development of more sophisticated devices (6).

Several companies produced stimulators. There are some variations between those instruments now on the market, some of which are discussed in a later section, but they all provide a portable means of electro-stimulation with variable wave form characteristics.

As one might expect, the acute and chronic pain states are the result of a wide spectrum of pathologic conditions, i.e., causalgia (8,9), polycythemia vera (10), peripheral nerve injury (11), phantom limb pain (12), lower back pain (13,14), bursitis (15), cervical pain (16,17), post herpetic neuralgia (18), cord injury (13), parturition (19), post-operative pain and ileus (20,21), and intractable cancer pain (22). Some of the patients treated with T.E.N.S. have reported a marked reduction of such pain. Many of the instances of T.E.N.S. success have been cited in the literature when used as a screening device before surgery or a first-line basis of treatment (22,23,24,25,26,27,28).

RECENT APPLICATIONS

The sensation of pain has been called an embarrassment to science (27). Today many Pain Control Centers (Figs. 2 & 3)

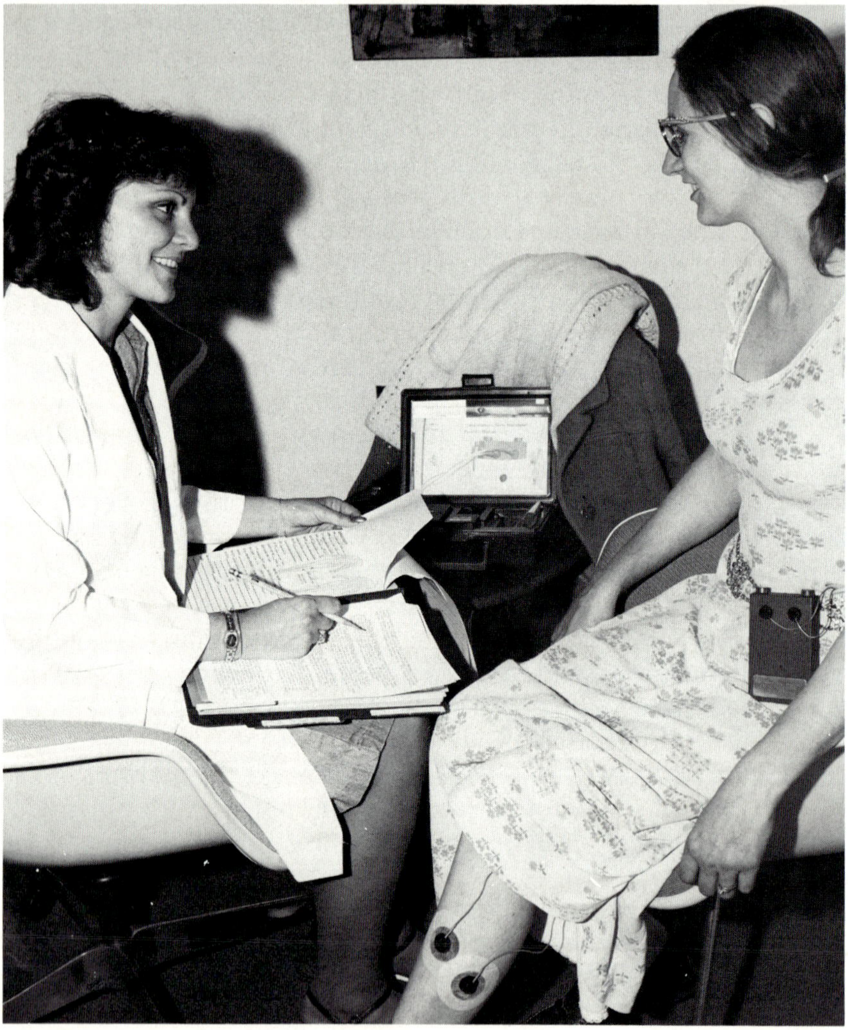

Figure 2. Counselling session during T.E.N.S. therapy in the Portland Control Center. Picture supplied by Electronic Research Devices.

employ electro-stimulation for the relief of intractable pain. Long (7) conducted a study of 200 pain patients during a one

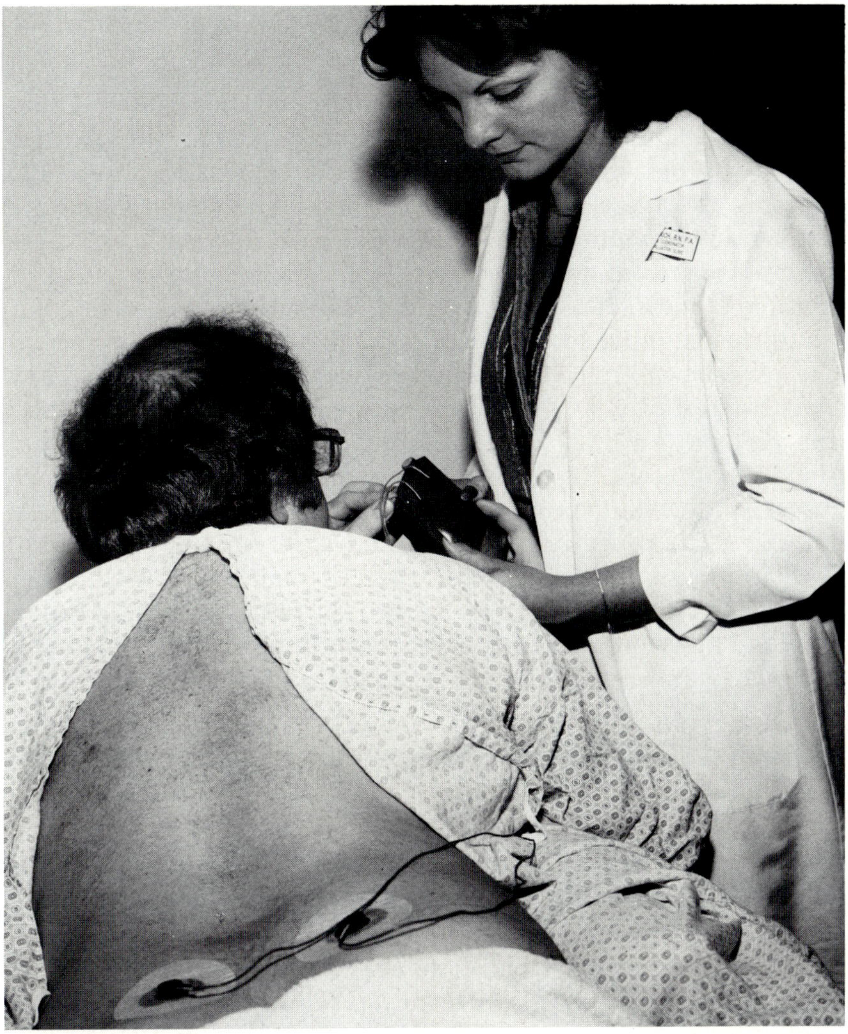

Figure 3. A patient treated for low back pain in the Portland Control Center. Picture supplied by Electronic Research Devices.

year period at the Pain Treatment Center at Johns Hopkins. They were on a specialty ward employing personnel skilled in pain treatment. By utilizing a program of increased activity, drug withdrawal, psychotropic medications and external stimulation, 70 percent of the patients obtained benefit from cutaneous stimulation compared with a 40 percent success ratio in a regular ward. The chief presenting problems were low back pain from degenerative disc disease complicated by arachnoiditis, chronic cervical disability from the same causes, and cancer or its sequela.

While at the University of Minnesota Pain Center, Long studied 400 pain patients, and attempted to determine to what extent the placebo effect influenced the results. Of these 400 patients, 203 were initially evaluated. About 150 patients were studied in the randomized sham system, the evaluation of these patients was abandoned, since the placebo effect was felt to be minimal. In all, 203 of the original 400 patients failed to complete the established protocol, or a small number experienced the placebo effect. Ultimately, 197 patients were used. They were treated by a single nurse, experienced in the utilization of the device. All had been failures in terms of conventional therapy, presenting serious pain problems. Of these, 78 reported excellent pain relief, 54 fair relief, and there were 62 failures (22,23). Failure was defined as a patient whose pain was under no better control than it had been with other therapeutic forms. There were also 20 patients in this group who had emotional problems which could have been considered as severe, and resulting from their pain states.

Long and Erickson felt that after using T.E.N.S. as a screening device prior to electrical implantation, if the use of external stimulation alone was a sufficient, a patient should be trained to use the device himself and allowed self-help by returning home with the unit, re-visiting the Pain Center for periodic re-evaluations by the physician and the team.

At the Sister Kenney Institute in Minneapolis, Burton (29) uses T.E.N.S. as a screening device to determine the degree of pain relief obtained and its duration following the cessation of stimulation. His experience indicates that this has a value as a screening tool, as well as being useful as a modality of therapy in its own right.

Clark (24) began working with implantable electrodes in Dallas in 1970. He has reported a declining number of patients receiving implanted dorsal column stimulation devices since, in his experience, T.E.N.S. is an alternative, non-invasive therapeutic device. Fifteen patients with chronic intractable pain needed no further therapy than T.E.N.S. It has produced 10 to 20 percent relief of chronic pain in patients he has seen, and has the additional value of safety and relative ease of patient use, without the risk of surgery which can still be performed at a later time.

Indeck (16) in Minnesota, admitted 40 patients to a Pain Ward and studied 50 patients in an out-patient clinic to determine the efficacy of T.E.N.S. He found that after the Gate Control Theory had been explained to the patients using the units, they would soon learn to find their own appropriate "trigger zones," impulse rates, intensity and frequency of application. If T.E.N.S. is initially successful for a patient, it generally remains so, although some of the efficacy may diminish in time. Indeck's Chapter discusses his findings more fully.

Picaza (30) in his analysis of 100 pain patients feels that, discounting the placebo effect, a significant number, possibly 50 percent, can be helped, while only about 10 percent experienced an increase in pain during or after the test stimulation. If the pain did increase, it usually did not continue beyond 24 hours. Even if it intensified this did not rule out the possibility of relief being obtained by changing stimulation parameters. His experience indicates, contrary to Wall and Sweet, that neither tingling nor stimulation of the coinciding nerve is essential for suppressing pain in some patients. While T.E.N.S. did not benefit all of his patients, in some cases in which it was beneficial, the effects were so dramatic that dubious patients were astonished. Some have continued to use it on an out-patient basis, or have purchased the units themselves.

At the Mayo Clinic, Ebersold (13) reporting a series of 230 patients receiving T.E.N.S., discovered 60 percent of them gaining some relief, eliminating the necessity for further surgery in those cases. He does not feel the relief was related exclusively to placebo or psychologic effects. 43 percent of the patients in this study purchased T.E.N.S. units, and, of those who did purchase the units, there seemed to be some slight decline of effectiveness of stimulation during follow-up.

Nielson, Adams, and Hosobuchi (31) of the University of California Medical Center now use T.E.N.S. for screening, rather than the previously used percutaneous dorsal column stimulation, to allow the patients to experience the expected stimulation paresthesias, and determine whether or not to proceed with surgery.

Shealy (15,19,32,33) at the Pain Rehabilitation Center, LaCrosse, Wisconsin, has published a great deal of work on the subject from its earliest developmental stages. In this book, he further delineates his experiences with the evolution of this method of pain control. In other works, he has reported that in cases where pain is focal, he can obtain 80 percent pain relief. The success ratio drops if the area of pain is more diffuse. In his presentation to the Congress of Neurosurgeons in Honolulu in 1973, he reviewed the steps taken to formulate the early stimulating devices, and continues to use T.E.N.S. in his treatment of acute pain. He considers it important in hastening of mobilization after abdominal, chest and hand surgery, and suggests a trial period with T.E.N.S. prior to any additional surgery for pain. To Shealy, one of its greatest assets is as a replacement for traditional pharmacologic pain therapy, with its attending side effects.

Kirsch (10,12), *et al.*, at the University of Colorado Medical Center, used Transcutaneous Electrical Neuro Stimulation for a variety of pain disorders in 56 patients, noting that 80 percent of them received brief relief, while over 25 percent secured relief over a long term period. They were particularly impressed by its usefullness in the management of such disorders as intractable itching secondary to polycythemia vera, and in some cases of post herpetic neuralgia and diabetic neuropathy.

Because of its safety and non-invasive nature, Hunt, Goodman and Bingham (34), Ohio State University College of Medicine, are refraining from further dorsal column stimulator implantations in favor of using T.E.N.S. as a trail.

Good to excellent results with T.E.N.S. used for patients suffering from acute pain resulting from such causes as carcinoma and arthritis involving neck, back and lumbar regions, were achieved by Winter (35) at the Hospital Center in Orange, New Jersey. His paper is brief, citing four case histories illustrative of the results achieved.

In addition to utilizing the modality for the above mentioned diseases, he has a study of 30 Multiple Sclerosis patients.

He describes these patients as having a deficiency relative to a chemical or electrical dysfunction. (Personal communication.) These patients are treated with T.E.N.S., with a biphasic square wave source. The electrodes were placed between the source of pathology and the spinal cord and brain. Minimal to moderate effect was noted when function was restored within 5 minutes. The unit of energy was a pulsed current source, adjustable for 0-76 MA measured into a 500 ohm load, and limited to a maximum of 100 volts. There was a reduction of spastic elements, and variable residual improvement after the cessation of stimulation. Normal function should result from the re-establishment of the deficient energy balance. The utilization of a biphasic square wave energy source is proposed as a potentially needed factor in multiple sclerosis and other neuromuscular disorders with this energy deficit.

Cauthen (11) in a study in Gainesville, Florida, reported on 113 patients who were referred to the University of Florida Division of Neurosurgery or to the Private Neurosurgical Service at the North Florida Regional Hospital at Gainesville. Most cases were related to lumbar spinal problems, cervical or thoracic nerve root injury, infections, or neoplasms. Additionally, there were peripheral nerve injuries and occipital neuralgia. All pains were of greater than six months duration. Most patients were on high doses of medication, and activity was significantly restricted. Nearly one-half of all patients in the group benefited from T.E.N.S. His conclusion is that T.E.N.S. is a safe and effective means of modifying the subjective sensation of pain.

In work done by Davis and Lentini (36), at the University of Miami, T.E.N.S. was deemed successful when pain reduction was sufficient to motivate the patient to continue wearing the device, and when there was at least a reduction in the analgesic drug dosage. Only 31 patients were studied, but in their findings, they note, according to the site of lesion, six successes, two partial successes, and eight failures, all in the conus, cauda, equina site. Five successes and six failures in the thoracic site were found, four cases - all failures in the cervical site of the lesion. They also comment that about two-thirds of the patients who were successfully treated had site of injury pain alone or in association with another type of pain. In their findings, root pain or phantom pain was not as easily treated, with only about one in five responding favorably to T.E.N.S.

Krainick *et al.* (37) at the University of Freiburg, West Germany, also found phantom pain only occasionally influenced by T.E.N.S. Localized stump pain responded better, but there was often difficulty in fitting the cutaneous electrode into the prosthesis. Work in achieving more adaptable electrodes is going on at present. If the patient had a local sensory loss, the possibility of cutaneous burning might occur. They, therefore, used T.E.N.S. as a screening device on all of their patients. If it was successful after two weeks of application, the patient was discharged with the device. Their patients, primarily war veterans whose pain has existed for years, had phantom pain, localized stump pain, and painful jerking of the stump as a spontaneous motor phenomena. If T.E.N.S. was not successful, the next step was the utilization of percutaneous stimulation of the spinal cord via special electrodes to simulate the postoperative situation.

Miles, of the Regional Neurological Center, Walton Hospital, Liverpool, England, includes a commentary on phantom pain in his section.

Starting with self made devices in the Clinic for Pain Relief and Surgical oncology in Gliwice, in Poland Rutkowski used electrical stimulation on 678 cases with the most encouraging results in neurological cases, ie.e., trigeminal neuralgia, as well as thoracic, cervical and bracial neuralgias. In a series of 83 cases, 35 good results were obtained, 34 fair, and 14 unsatisfactory. The best responses were in people of less than 50 years of age. Rutkowski, in his section, also discusses the headache problem, wherein male response was much greater than female, while there was little overall response in the rheumatic diseases. It must be noted that in this clinic, their preference in primary usage was by means of insertion of needle electrodes rather than the cutaneous electrodes which we have been discussing previously (38).

Kurzbauer, also from Poland, treats the efficacy of T.E.N.S. in dealing with the problem of varicose ulcers in one section, and post-operative pain and ileus, in another chapter. This topic is also examined by VanderArk of Denver, Colorado.

Nathan and Wall (18) in London's National Hospital for Nervous Disorders, treated two groups of patients. Nine had attended the hospital for two to seven years, 21 had attended for one to three years. All other forms of therapy for post herpetic neuralgia had failed for the entire group of 30 patients. Group 1 (nine patients) was treated first by spraying the skin with ethyl chloride spray, using vibrators, secondly percutaneous stimulation, and thirdly - Transcutaneous Electrical Neuro Stimulation for as long as they desired. This could be for 12 hours or more, if they wished, daily. At first, placement of the electrodes away from the area of skin tenderness where the skin was markedly hyperesthetic and hyperanalgesic, was necessary.

Nathan and Wall postulated that the tingling sensation caused tactile paresthesia replacing the pain sensation. The patients were asked to keep records of their pain and medication dosages. On those with good results, the medication dosages declined. In all, 16 patients had some relief - six with total, seven moderate, three slight. Of the six with total improvement, when the stimulation was discontinued, the pain worsened. When stimulation was begun again, lessening of pain became apparent. However, in eight cases, the neuralgia gradually continued to improve. Their findings indicate that those with the most severe neuralgic pain do not get relief. Other complaints were the necessity of carrying the apparatus and wearing of the electrodes. Also, some old people are afraid of electricity. In addition, there was some patient disappointment, as they had hoped for a *cure* rather than pain alleviation.

Schuster, of the International Pain Control Center, Silver Springs, Maryland, will examine the center's success utilizing drug reduction, increased movement, close physician and nurse supervision, rather than patient percentile responses to gauge progress relative to individual pain states. In this out-patient center, T.E.N.S., along with exercise, medication, and a strongly positive attitude on the part of the nursing and ancillary personnel involved in patient care, have combined to produce relief in 80 percent of their cases, with the greatest success with low back and cervical pain. In his Chapter, he cites a number of case histories, and the outcome after T.E.N.S. as a major part of rehabilitive therapy.

Lampe, a Registered Physical Therapist in Kansas City, Missouri, finds his patients - all referrals from physicians in the area - receiving 60 to 70 percent pain relief. In his Chapter he discusses the role of the physical therapist, as well as the fear, skepticism, and reluctance to try a new form of therapy which he encounters in some patients.

EFFICACY OF T.E.N.S.

The brief summation of the history of the development of electro-analgesia, and the studies cited here from a variety of institutions world-wide, imply pain relief has been obtained wholly, or in part, for a number of divergent conditions. Over the years, various wave forms, frequencies, currents and voltage combinations have been tried, and more than 2000 patients have been reported benefiting from T.E.N.S. (5,8,15,16,28).

Although some sharp pain and referred hyperalgia may be increased (16,17,18,30) and interferences with EEG, ECG, (17) or demand type cardiac pacemakers must be considered (35), these are minor considerations to be weighed against the potential gain from the treatments.

Additionally, some patients become "addicted" to their stimulators, but this does not seem to lead to psychological dependence or difficulty in withdrawal (17).

There are occasional allergic reactions which have been reported from contact with electrodes, but different electrodes and gels are being developed to minimize this problem (23).

Pain is a subjective phenomenon and the relief of pain is a private sensation whose quality is known only to the patient. Therefore, many of the studies allow the patient to serve as his own control in determining his state of comfort.

After a diagnostic work-up and the determination of a course of therapy, the relief of pain becomes an important obligation of all physicians. Suffering has an extremely debilitating effect on patients, causing significant lost man-hours from work, personality problems for the individual and his familial interaction. Therefore, the alleviation of pain and its consequences are of significant importance to all physicians.

Having traced the development of electroanalgesia, concentrating on the specificity of T.E.N.S. as a non pharmacologic, non-invasive, non-toxic adjunct to other modalities of pain therapy, we will examine in greater detail its current utilization, studying areas in which it is proving itself of great value in a variety of acute and chronic pain states.

BIBLIOGRAPHY

1. Bonica, J.: Preface, *Adv. in Neurol.* Int. Symposium of Pain Vol. *4*, vii-x, Raven Press, New York, 1975
2. Stillings, D.: A Survey of the History of Electrical Stimulation for Pain to 1900. *Med. Instrum., 9*:(6) 255-9. Nov.-Dec., 1975.
3. Melzack, R., Wall, P.: Pain Mechanisms: A New Theory. *Science, 150:*971-973, 1965.
4. Wall, P. and Sweet, W.: Temporary Abolition of Pain in Man. *Science,155*:108, 1967.
5. Sweet, W. H., Wepsic, J. G.: Treatment of Chronic Pain by Stimulation of Fibers of Primary Afferent Neuron. *Trans. Am. Neurol. Assn.,93*:103-6, 1968.
6. Sweet, W. H. and Wepsic, J.G.: Stimulation of the Posterior Columns of the Spinal Cord for Pain Control: Indications, Techniques, Results. *Clin, Neurosurg.*, 278-310. Proceedings of the College of Neurosurgeons, Honolulu, 1973, Williams and Wilkins, 1974.
7. Long, D. M.: Use of Cutaneous Afferent Stimulation of the Context of a Chronic Pain Treatment Center. Abstract of the 7th Annual Meeting of Neuroelectric Soc., New Orleans, La., p. 52, Nov. 20-23, 1974.
8. Sternschein, M. J., Myers, S. J., Frewin, D. B., Downey, J. A.: Causalgia. *Arch. Phys. Med. Rehabil.,56*:58-63, Feb., 1975.
9. Mayer, G. A., Fields, H. L.: Causalgia Treated by Selected Large Fibrous Stimulation of Peripheral Nerve. *Brain,95*:163, 1972.
10. Kirsch, W. D.: A New Method of Managing Chronic Pain. *Med. Times,102*(11) 115-118, Nov., 1974.
11. Cauthen, J. C., Renner, E. J.: Transcutaneous and Peripheral Nerve Stimulation for Chronic Pain States. *Surg. Neurol.,4*:102-104, July, 1975.
12. Kirsch, W. D., Lewis, J., Simon, R.: Experiences With Electrical Stimulation Devices for Control of Pain. *Med. Instrum.,9*(5) 217-20, Sept.-Oct., 1975.
13. Ebersold, M., Laws, E., Stonnington, H., Stillwell, G.: Transcutaneous Electrical Stimulation for Treatment of Chronic Pain, a Preliminary Report. *Surg. Neurol.,4*:96-99, July, 1975.
14. Ersek, R. A.: Low Back Pain, Prompt Relief with Transcutaneous Neuro-Stimulation. *Orthopaedic Review,* Vol. 5 *12:*27-31 Dec. 76.
15. Shealy, C. N., Maurer, D.: Transcutaneous Nerve Stimulation for Control of Pain. *Surg. Neurol.,2*:45-47, Jan., 1974.
16. Indeck, W., Printy, A.: Skin Application of Electrical Impulses for Relief of Pain in Chronic Orthopaedic Conditions. *Minn. Med.,*305-9, April, 1975.
17. Loeser, J. D., Black, R. G., Christman, A.: Relief of Pain by Transcutaneous Neuro-Stimulation. *J. Neurosurg.,42*:308-14, March, 1975.
18. Nathan, P. W., Wall, P. D.: Treatment of Post-Herpetic Neuralgia by Prolonged Electrical Stimulation. *Brit. Med. J., 3:*645-7, Sept., 1974.
19. Shealy, C. N.: The Viability of the External Electrical Stimulation as a Therapeutic Modality. *Med. Instrum.,9*(5):211-12, Sept.-Oct., 1975.
20. Hymes, A. C.: *Treatment of Post-Op Ileus.* Presentation to American College of Surgeons, Miami, Florida, October, 1974.
21. Vander Ark, J. D., Mc Grath, K. A.: Transcutaneous Electrical Stimulation in the Treatment of Postoperative Pain. *Am. J. Surg.,130*:338-40, Sept., 1975.
22. Long, D. M.: Cutaneous Afferent Stimulation for Relief of Chronic Pain. *Clin. Neurosurg.* Proceedings of Congress of Neurological Surgeons, Honolulu, 1973. 255-267 Williams and Wilkins, 1974.

23. Long, D. M.: External Electrical Stimulation as a Treatment of Chronic Pain. *Minn. Med.,57*(3):195-198, March, 1974.

24. Clark, K.: Electrical Stimulation of the Nervous System for Control of Pain. University of Texas Southwestern Medical School Experience. *Surg. Neurol.,4*:164-166, July, 1975.

25. Screening Procedure Relieves Chronic Pain. *J.A.M.A.,223*(9):968-9, Feb. 26, 1973.

26. Davis, R., Lentini, R.: Transcutaneous Nerve Stimulation for Treatment of Pain in Spinal Cord Injured Patients. *Bull. Prosth. Res.*,298-301, Fall, 1974.

27. Ferguson, V., Barkdoll, D.: Pain and its Alleviation: Summary of a Forum. *Arch. Phys. Med. Rehabil.,56*:172-3, April, 1975.

28. Long, D. M., Erickson, D.: Stimulation of the Posterior Columns of the Spinal Cord for Relief of Intractable Pain. *Surg. Neurol,4*:134-141, July, 1975.

29. Burton, C.: Dorsal Column Stimulation: Optimization of Application. *Surg. Neurol.,4*:171-179, July, 1975.

30. Picaza, J., Cannon, D., Hunter, S., Boyd, A., Guma, J., Maurer, D.: Pain Suppression by Peripheral Nerve Stimulation, Part I: Observations with Transcutaneous Stimuli. *Surg. Neurol.,4*:105-114, July, 1975.

31. Nielson, K., Adams, J., Hosobuchi, Y.: Experience with Dorsal Column Stimulation for the Relief of Chronic Intractable Pain: 1968-1973. *Surg. Neurol.,4*:148-152, July, 1975.

32. Shealy, C. N.: Transcutaneous Electrical Stimulation for Control of Pain. *Clin. Neurosurg.,* Proceedings of Congress of Neurological Surgeons, Honolulu, 1973. 269-277, Williams and Wilkins, 1974.

33. Shealy, C. N.: Dorsal Column Stimulation: Optimization of Application. *Surg. Neurol.,4*:142-145, July, 1975.

34. Hunt, W., Goodman, J., Bingham, W.: Stimulation of the Dorsal Spinal Cord for Treatment of Intractable Pain: A Preliminary Report. *Surg. Neurol.,4*:153-156, July, 1975.

35. Winter, A.: Pain Relief-Transcutaneous Neuro-Stimulation. *J. Med. Sco. N. Jer.,71*(5):365-367, May, 1974.

36. Davis, R., Lentini, R.: Transcutaneous Nerve Stimulation for Treatment of Pain in Patients with Spinal Cord Injury. *Surg. Neurol.,4*:100-101, July, 1975.

37. Krainick, K., Thoden, U., Riechert, T.: Spinal Cord Stimulation in Post Amputation Pain. *Surg. Neurol, 4:*167-170, July, 1975.

38. Rutowski, B., Niedzialkowska, T., Otto, J.: *Electro-stimulation in the Management of Chronic Pain.* Springer-Verlag. pp. 457-460, 1975.

39. Howson, David C.: Peripheral Neural Excitability, Implications for Transcutaneous Electrical Nerve Stimulation, *Physical Therapy., 58:* 1467-1473, Dec., 1978.

40. Hamer, Debra, and Howson, David C.: Bibliography on Electroanalgesia. *Physical Therapy, 58* (12), 1485-1492, Dec., 1978.

Chapter 2

THE PSYCHOLOGICAL ASPECTS OF PAIN RELATIVE TO THE EFFICACY OF T.E.N.S.

ALAN V. BORNSTEIN, Ph.D.

The dilemma of evaluating the pain patient relative to establishment of an initiation of therapy is a puzzlement to many in the medical profession. We seek to analyze pain, striving for therapeutic consistency and efficacy. (1)

Regardless of the type of pain, one of the most prevalent questions asked prior to any treatment is "Is this individual's pain functional, organic, or a combination of both?" With the exception of acute pain stemming from physical trauma of recent origin, most pain is both functional and organic. We have not yet seen a case of "chronic intractable pain" without a psychological overlay, no matter how clearly its organic etiology is demonstrated.

Treatment modalities may differ according to the answer to the functional versus organic question. And there immediately follows another query: "What percentage of each (i.e., functional or organic) is involved?" With the possible exception of some good promise and to this time rather weak research results, in the opinion of the clinician demanding an easy answer, we remain held to some rather lengthy procedures to seek answers.

As a clinical psychologist specializing in reduction of functional and organic pain, it is possibly a fortuitous fact that my office is deemed the "office of last resort." As a "last resort" consultant, I generally have a plethora of information about the new patient. The usefulness of this data will, for now, remain questionable. However, virtually all the patients have had a complete history and physical and probably have been to 15 or 20 physicians, and have, at their disposal a portion of the United States Pharmacopaea either in their purse or medicine cabinet.

The first visit to my office consists of a routine, if detailed, psychiatric type history incorporating some germane physical history as well. During the information-gathering session, the procedures for the next steps are outlined, sometimes to the distress of the patient, some of whom have the lurking feeling of being in a witch doctor's office, and half expect an on-the-spot, magical cure.

The next step is psychological testing, using two main instruments, one well known to almost everyone working in this field. The Minnesota Multiphasic Personality Inventory, or M.M.P.I., and the Pain Apperception Test or P.A.T. by Petrovich, published by Western Psychological Services of California. Roche Psychiatric Services Institute provides a computer scored version of the M.M.P.I. to psychologists and physicians. This consists of 550 true/false questions. On the basis of the patient's answers, a three to six page print-out is computer generated. Aside from the obvious help this anecdotal portion of the print-out presents, a closer look at the patient's clinical scales for patterns may afford a working hypothesis as to the possible efficacy of treatment. There are a number of important scales which should be specifically mentioned. First are the validity or "lie" scales. These actually measure test taking results, can provide obvious important diagnostic clues to the patient's personality, and chances of success in treatment.

We next have four essential scales meriting discussion relative to pain diagnosis and management. These four are: Hs (Hypochondriasis), D (Depression), Hy (Hysteria), Pd)Psychopathic Deviate), Sternbach (2) notes that "different scale configurations, as well as absolute scale scores, carry different diagnostic implications." Generally, diagnosis depends on an overall configuration of scores, but the highest scale score is most likely to indicate the individual's self perceived complaints. It should be noted that many of the indicators and scale interrelationships have not been statistically cross validated on control subjects, and are only suggestive. They have been found helpful on an empiric basis.

If a profile indicates the highest score to be on the Hypochondriasis scale, this presents a number of possible inferences. The first indication is that the patient is preoccupied with somatic problems to the extreme. He probably has a wide range and variety of body ailments including many which are totally unrelated to his actual pain. If other high scores are found to be Depression and Hysteria, there seems to be a relatively poor success potential in treatment of this patient. One reason is that Hypochondriacal patients cannot seem to ignore any of their pains, no matter how slight (3). They exist on pain and, in fact, may utilize pain as a mechanism to keep them from decompensating. There may be valid question as to whether these patients should be worked with in the absence of ongoing psychotherapy and/or psychotropic medication.

Depression as the major or highest clinical scale is the second most commonly found and crucial profile. It is important to recognize that these are more reactive or exogenous rather than endogenous depressions. Many of these patients realize that they are in the midst of a vicious cycle and that, while pain of organic etiology may have caused their depression initially, the depression itself may reinforce and exacerbate the pain. Here anti-depressant medication may be of great use as an adjunct to T.E.N.S. treatments. Patients who have this profile of Reactive Depression on the M.M.P.I. have been shown to be very amenable to treatment, and seem less likely to develop other somatic problems of psychogenic etiology in the post-treatment phase.

The third profile commonly found has been called the Somatization Reaction by Sternbach. In this profile, one typically finds elevated Hysterial and Hypochondrical scores, with a somewhat lower Depression score. This profile has long been associated with somatic complaints in psychiatric patients. This type patient preoccupies himself with somatic concerns. At the same time he denies, on a psychologically hysterical basis, any emotional problems, including depression, which is most commonly repressed. Hence it scores lower on the clinical scales than either Hypochondria or Hysteria. There is good reason to assume that this type of patient uses his physical symptoms as a defense against his latent depression, which can be avoided as long as the somatic symptoms persist. This mechanism of dealing with pain is common in both psychogenic and somatogenic patients. It does differ from the Hypochondriacal patient who constantly replaces old symptoms with new ones, without doing anything about any of them. In this Somatization Reaction, the patient typically concentrates on one single pain symptom, almost exclusively, and does not have a "generalized body pain reaction." Patients with this profile generally do fairly well in pain communities or pain treatment programs.

The fourth commonly found profile deals with the "manipulator." This profile has typically elevated (above 70) scales on all four areas under discussion: Hysteria, Hypochondrical, Depressive, and Psychopathic Deviate. Their surgical histories are longer, more complicated, more frequent, and less necessary. This type of individual can and generally does persuade his various and sundry physicians to write unnecessary prescriptions, perform unnecessary operations, and sign disability forms until there is an epidemic of writers' cramp among all his physicians. This is not to say that these manipulators are malingerers. Many have legitimate organic findings, but strong as these symptoms may be, and hard as the evidence may be, this type of person will use his symptoms both consciously and deliberately to achieve any and all of his goals. The "typical" low back patient may sometimes fall into this category, although not invariably. This profile sounds very bleak, at least for treatment prospects, but fortunately it is not as common as it seems, although treating only one of these patients may seem like one hundred. If they don't work well in a program, they should be excluded, especially in group therapy sessions, because this type of patient may destroy a pain milieu group.

The functional utility of the M.M.P.I. can be seen. I find it an extremely useful instrument for screening chronic pain patients, prior to T.E.N.S. or any other therapy is contemplated.

The other instrument, or test, mentioned earlier is the Pain Apperception Test, or P.A.T. This, with appropriate, simple instructions, is basically self-administered, and not terribly stressful or threatening to patients. The P.A.T. consists of 25 individual pictures, divided into three major segments. The first nine pictures illustrate felt pain sensations. The next eight - divided into pairs, deal with anticipation of pain versus felt sensation of pain. The final series deals with the origin of the pain sensation; that is whether the pain is self-inflicted, or inflicted by others.

As the patient examines each picture, he is required to answer two questions about it. The first is "How does the man feel?" The second - "How long will it hurt him?" These are rated on a 1-7 scale, with the results being interpreted for a) intensity or sensitivity to felt pain of one's self, b) duration or the tendency to experience pain over longer or shorter time periods, and c) intensity plus duration, or overall pain sensitivity.

The higher the score on the test, the more sensitive the individual is to pain. In other words, low thresholds for pain generate high scores on this test, while high thresholds to pain will generate a lower score.

These two tests, the M.M.P.I. and P.A.T., along with the initial clinical or psychiatric interview sessions provide a relatively sound screening technique, considering the obvious limitations of any psychological testing.

I feel the screening techniques tend to enhance the effects of T.E.N.S. because it places an "I care" feeling between clinician and patient. This can and should be communicated to the patient in a session when test results are interpreted to him, and a plan for treatment is agreed upon. This plan is a necessary and sometimes a negotiable commodity. If, as a treating person, you are not getting full cooperation from your patient, then T.E.N.S. or any other modality will be all but useless. Many times the post-test or post-screening discussion ends in a verbal contract. This contract or agreement involves making explicit what has probably been implicit previously. The patient has to verbalize his desire to modify his pain, and his intention to work very hard at doing so. The treating person must be frank and open in giving the patient realistic goals and methods of therapy. This give-and-take session must be handled positively and assertively if we wish to maximize our chances of success.

Screening procedures do not insure automatic success.

When working with T.E.N.S. or other pain reduction techniques, the personal touch enhances the potential outcome of the therapy. I have seen noticeable differences in the effectiveness of T.E.N.S. done personally and consistantly in my office, and the same treatment carried out by a succession of treating persons in a hospital or clinic situation. It spite of the perceptible differences T.E.N.S. therapy is not as affected as are other treatment modalities such as hypnosis or biofeedback.

My experience shows, for chronic or acute pain of demonstrable organic etiology, T.E.N.S. offers the most rapid, inoffensive, and in general the most effective method for pain suppression. My associate and I have used T.E.N.S. on approximately 100 patients. Certain patterns and tendencies toward limited predictability are emerging. It is possible that our office, providing both psychological and psychiatric services, is one of the few out-patient facilities combining this speciality with T.E.N.S. for the reduction of pain. Emotional distress is intimately related to many types of pain such as migraine and migrainous headaches, tension headaches, low back pain, etc.

In my experience there have been numerous startling successes, using T.E.N.S., and startling failures as well. Almost all the patients have been physician referred; the vast majority by neurosurgeons. As a result, I have had much more exposure to migraine and migrainous headaches, cervical strain, and low back problems with sciatic pain, than I have with the arthritic problem or post trauma pain. This exposure is changing because of the development within our local community hospital of a Pain Community. Additionally, entities such as labyrinthitis, trigeminal neuralgia, and temporomandibular joint pain have proven to be amenable to T.E.N.S., from my experience.

Temporomandibular joint pain (TMJ) is an excruciating pain syndrome. Recently many conscientious dentists have been made aware of their role in the treatment of this malady and the importance of proper jaw alignment which can alleviate much of the pain This is not as simple a procedure as it sounds, but nevertheless, it points out the paramount role a well prepared dentist can and should play in this problem. I have been working for the last 18 months with 12 patients with this disease. T.E.N.S. has been gratifyingly successful in reducing the pain about 80% of the time. The dentist with whom I work on this syndrome was so excited about T.E.N.S. that he now has a machine in each examining room. He reports about the same level of success in pain reduction as I have found in my office. So far surgery has been avoided using T.E.N.S. and careful dentistry in all 12 of the TMJ patients we have been treating.

The results achieved with migraine headache patients have also been exciting. Prior to my experience with TENS, a referral in my office of a migraine headache patient was like the "voice of doom." The only ammunition I had going for me was hypnosis, which was not very successful in migraine therapy. Since my office is generally considered the last resort, most of these patients presenting have been on Ergotamine or one of the derivatives for many years, with little or no relief. With the use of T.E.N.S., I have had about 70% success in aborting a migraine headache in about 20 minutes time. This procedure becomes more viable and successful as the patients work by themselves, utilizing their own device at home. Numerous calls from patients who have been prescribed the T.E.N.S. machine for home use confirm its efficacy in migraine headache treatment. This gives treating persons a tremendous edge on this problem. Patients can be told more positively that there is a viable alternative to the medication, and in addition, perhaps for the first time, good promise of a technique which will stop a migraine headache already in progress. Of equal importance is the fact that these patients will be able to comfortably continue a normal days' activities. The use of T.E.N.S. in these cases avoids numerous office visits, emergency room trips, and may eliminate much of the narcotic analgesics necessary to relieve the pain of migrainous headaches.

There seem to be some important differences, in my experience, in the effectiveness of T.E.N.S. in acute versus chronic cervical strain. Chronic cervical strains, although amenable to T.E.N.S. have not been as consistently relieved (at least on an outpatient basis) as acute cervical strains. I am sure the length of time between injury and treatment has much to do with the efficacy of any therapeutic modality. Another fact to consider is that in certain cases the pain remains because many of these patients are involved in litigation and compensation cases. The secondary gains they are receiving may outweigh the possibilities for pain relief. The area involving compensation and litigation cases frequently renders any treatment modality including T.E.N.S. ineffective. This is not to say that these patients are not experiencing genuine pain. But most tend to hang on to it with the tenacity of a bulldog. . . . .at least until after a settlement, at which time they are willing to become real patients. As mentioned earlier, these patients can be detected using good screening techniques at the time of psychological testing, at which time we may become aware of the types of profiles which may indicate possible lack of success (4). Naturally, any individual with a profile indicating possible lack of success should not automatically be eliminated from the treatment program, but I have found that the more information available prior to treatment, the greater will be the potential therapy's chances for success (5).

In addition to my treatment of patients presenting with migraine, cervical strain, low back pain or TMJ, I have had some excellent results with cases involving acute post herpetic neuralgia or post herpetic neuropathy. Usually these patients seen in my office have been on many types of medication, prior to referral, with minimal or no results. Until the practicality and efficacy of T.E.N.S. had been established, the most common combination of medication for these patients had been Amytriptyline 75 mg. H.S and Fluphenazine 1 mg. T.I.D. My treatment of post herpetic neuropathy has been extremely limited. Of the four patients with whom I have worked, three received immediate relief after an initial 15 minute exposure to T.E.N.S. Times of relief varied from 3 to 8 hours, and relief appeared to increase as the T.E.N.S. treatments were continued. As the patients began using the machine, they found the length of time of relief was more prolonged.

In summary, I have found that, through careful psychological screening, a good majority of my patients have shown significant benefits from the use of T.E.N.S. as measured by pain relief and decrease of medication. I consider T.E.N.S. an extremely important part of my private practice and have already started to institute the incorporation of this therapeutic modality in the pain community at my local hospital. Here as well as in my private practice, T.E.N.S. will play a vital role.

BIBLIOGRAPHY

1. Gooddy, W: On the Nature of Pain; Brain, J. *of Neuros* 53:118-31, 1957
2. Sternbach, R.A.: *Pain Patients; Traits and Treatment.* New York, New York Academic Press 1974.
3. Shealy, C.N., Maurer, D.: Transcutaneous Nerve stimulation for control of pain: a preliminary technical note *Surg. Neurol.,*2:45-7, Jan. 1974
4. Sternbach, R.: Evaluation of Pain Relief *Surg. Neurol.,*4:199-201, Jul. 1975
5. Fordyce, W.E., Fowler, R.S., Lehmann, J.F., DeLateur, B.J.: Some implications of learning in problems of chronic pain. *J. Chronic Dis.,*21:179-190, 1968.

Chapter 3

THE OPERATION OF A PAIN CONTROL CENTER, ITS ESTABLISHMENT AND IMPORTANCE IN THE MEDICAL COMMUNITY

GERALD D. SCHUSTER, MD., and

ESTELLE KORNHAUSER, R.N.

Our Pain Control Center, and those similar in nature which have developed over the past few years, are dedicated to the *patient*. His pain and related problems are the primary concern of the staff - both the nursing and paramedical personnel.

Staff selection for such a Pain Center must seek nurses who know and understand pain, and consequently are able to relate to the patient with empathy, compassion and understanding. The patient is in an environment where there is total concern for the relief or management of his pain and the accompanying personal and physical problems.

Control or modulation of pain has always been at the forefront of medicine. Most attempts to control this thalmic oriented sensation have been aimed directly at that center, to either dull perception or increase one's threshold to tolerate the pain entity.

Various attempts at control via external stimulation or

means such as emollients, rubefacients, anesthetic agents, galvanic stimulation, machines to deliver "deep" warmth - infrared, diathermy, and ultrasound have been tried, with varying results.

Only in the past few years have several manufacturing companies developed machines which could deliver a standardized stimulus perceived only by the "A" sensory fibers, allowing us to pursue the use of a more scientific and reproduceable external pain control mechanism. The "C" fibers in apparent accordance with Melzack and Wall's Gate Control Theory (Chapters 1,4,16), permits us to treat patients suffering with both acute and chronic musculoskeletal pain with a high degree of success.

Because of the increasing interest in the management of pain in centers specifically designed for this purpose, many physicians have been studying the effects and benefits of Transcutaneous Electrical Neuro Stimulation on their chronic pain patients.

The efficacy of T.E.N.S. in the more serious chronic syndromes has led us to use it in the acute pain states associated with various musculoskeletal injuries. The common denominator to successful pain control with this modality has been the individual administration or instruction in its usage.

We soon learned that many of the "failures" in treatment of our patient population were not the fault of the patient or the machine. Lack of understanding on the part of the patient as to how, when, and where to use the appliance, and what was to be expected of it, caused misunderstandings which we were able to rectify.

In order to circumvent this problem, we trained a nurse to work with the patients who were to use T.E.N.S. as part of their therapy. Shortly after she began working with these patients, it became obvious she would not be able to carry on her other functions within the office. It was at this time that the establishment of a separate out-patient pain control center emerged from concept to reality.

Our center was set up as a referral facility to handle the needs present in our medical community. Unless an individual physician is willing to have his nurse, paramedic, or himself specially trained to administer to this type of patient, with this form of therapy, the plan is doomed to failure before its beginning. Our nursing and therapy staff are dedicated to trying to modulate or alleviate pain as the patient is recuperating from musculoskeletal injury, and being taught to rehabilitate himself physically and psychologically.

The staff has been specially trained not only in the use of the particular T.E.N.S. unit we have found most suited to our needs, but also in rehabilitative and therapeutic exercises. The treatment becomes quite personal, and the staff is advised to spend part of each one-hour treatment session talking with the patient about any special problems which may have arisen, thus dealing with difficulties at an early stage.

Those patients who have initially been seen at the center, then given devices to be used at home have frequent telephone follow-ups. They are advised to return at least on a monthly basis so that their progress may be checked and any changes in electrode placement or duration of time for utilization of the device may be altered.

The patient who has complete freedom of changing leads without supervision soon falls into a typical pattern of change and ultimately experiences poor results from use of the machine.

CLINIC SET-UP

Each of our four treatment rooms has been set up in similar fashion. The decor is plain and pleasant. Our receptionist-secretary handles all administrative problems concerning the visit and the T.E.N.S. units, thus freeing our nurses to deal strictly with the patients' pain problems.

Since our patients have been referred by a physician, their clinical diagnoses are known. We request the treating physician send a brief clinical summary. (Figure 1)

The nurse then formulates a more complete history and evaluation for the possible benefits from T.E.N.S. These are noted on the anatomical sketch. (Figure 2).

Some pain syndromes will not respond to T.E.N.S. Patients with these conditions are appraised of the situation and advised to reconsult their own physician.

Once the patient has been evaluated and the usual infor-

DOCTORS REFERRAL FORM

DOCTOR: ____________________

ADDRESS: ____________________

TELEPHONE: ____________________

PATIENTS NAME: ____________________

MEDICAL HISTORY:

SYMPTONS AT PRESENT TIME:

DOCTORS ORDERS - TNS POINTS:

MEDICATIONS:

EXERCISES:

REMARKS:

Figure 1.

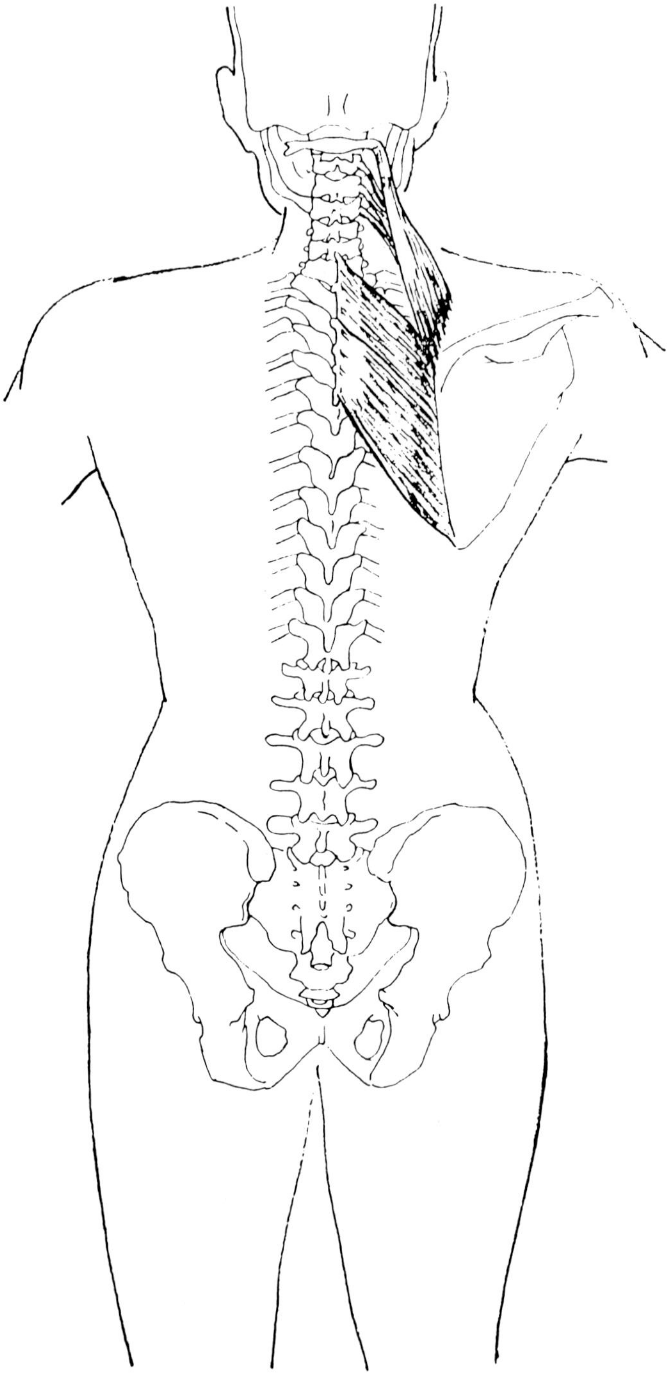

Figure 2.

mation charted, we also keep visual records on one of our anatomical charts to assure accurate placement and replacement of electrodes on subsequent visits.

On the introductary visit any fears the patient may have concerning "electric shock," "burns," "pain" or other areas of uneasiness are dealt with calmly by showing the patient the manner in which the machine works, and instructing him in some of the theory behind it. The more informed patient is better to cope with and assist in treatment. The patient is also given a brief trial with the device at this time.

On subsequent visits to the center, which are necessary in order to make certain there is, in fact, a beneficial result, the patients are questioned, treated, and taught exercises indicated for the pathology presented.

When a patient's pain is lessened, cooperation in a rehabilitative program increases, and a security in the belief of the treatment undergone is established.

The initial placement of the electrodes may not be the ultimate site. Patients may respond to electrode placement at a painful site along the course of a nerve or at the more central origin of that nerve. They will sometimes respond only when more than one area is treated, although one site may be far removed from the other.

Several visits may be necessary before deciding whether or not a given patient will respond better to treatments given only in the center, or continue with further utilization of a T.E.N.S. machine at home.

The following case histories will illustrate the types of patients who come to our center from referring physicians for treatment.

CASE HISTORY 1: Diagnosis: Severe Adhesive Capsulitis

The patient is a 51 year old white female who had complaints of a painful left shoulder and arm for 2 years. She had noted the onset of pain 6-7 weeks prior to her visit to her physician. The area was injected with cortisone with no apparent relief. She was referred to an orthopaedic surgeon, who made a provisional diagnosis following x-rays of the shoulder: severe adhesive capsulitis.

Manipulation of the left shoulder was done under general anesthesia. The patient's range of motion had improved well following surgery. Eight months later she began complaining of increased pain and difficulties with the right shoulder. A diagnosis of early adhesive capsulitis was made. After treatment of injections of cortisone into the rotator cuff and physical therapy treatments, it was decided that manipulation of the right shoulder was necessary. This was performed.

Because of considerable pain and restriction of motion over the right greater tuberosity, she was started on T.E.N.S. treatments. The patient appeared to respond well to treatments and began to utilize the unit at home. She continued with therapy at home for three months. Then she returned the device since she was free of pain and had complete mobility of her arm (Fig. 3).

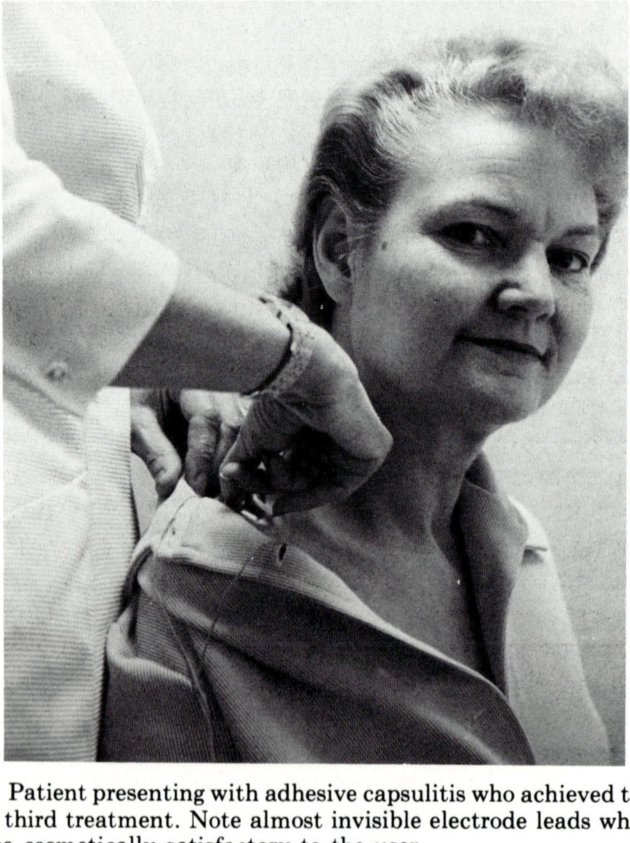

Figure 3. Patient presenting with adhesive capsulitis who achieved total relief after the third treatment. Note almost invisible electrode leads which make the device cosmetically satisfactory to the user.

CASE HISTORY 2: Diagnosis: Diabetic neuropathy

The patient is a white male, age 50. He stated he had had no sensation in extremities for the past eight years.

Medications: Apresoline 10 mg qid
NPH Insulin 80 u qd
Atromid S 500 mg qid
Tegretol (with poor response)

The electrodes were placed at the ulnar and radial nerve sites on the right and left wrists. The patient had immediate sensation in fingers, and hands were warm to touch.

He was checked regularly by telephone and continued to have good response to T.E.N.S., was able to drive a car. The results pleased him greatly.

When seen in the office 6 months later, the patient felt he was having less success with T.E.N.S. Electrodes were placed at the ulnar and radial nerves below the elbow at the right and left arms. He had immediate sensation to his fingers. Fingers felt warm to touch and color improved.

This particular patient uses the device continuously in order to maintain sensation and pain relief. (Constant usage is necessary in a small percentage of patients.)

CASE HISTORY 3: Diagnosis: Lateral and Medial Epicondylitis

The patient is a 42 year old white female who presented herself with complaints of pain not related to known trauma. The area of pain was in the right elbow, with increasing pain in pressure directly over the lateral epicondylar area and down into the brachial radialis muscle mass.

She was sent to the pain center for treatment with T.E.N.S. Electrodes were placed at the epicondylar origin, approximately one and one-half inch below the area on the muscle mass of the medial radialis, mid-portion of the dorsal aspect of the area along the brachial radialis, mid-portion of the dorsal aspect of the area along the brachial radialis, and at the dorsal aspect of the wrist.

The patient responded well on the first treatment, and was able to extend her elbow without pain. She was anxious to use the instrument at home, and continued to do so with excellent response. Her exercise program was also continued, and she was pleased with the treatment.

CASE HISTORY 4: Diagnosis: Chronic Plantar Fasciatis and Calcaneal Spur - Right Foot

Patient is a white female, age 50, first seen in 1969. She was treated conservatively with medications and injections to the painful site. Butazolidin Alka was prescribed.

July - SX procedure of plantar fasciectomy and removal of calcaneal spur on right foot. The patient continued to improve following this procedure, wearing molded arch supports.

March, 3 years later. The patient presented herself with acute chest and back pain. Cardiac problems were ruled out, and a diagnosis of costotransverse facet syndrome was noted. The patient started on colbenamid.

February, 1 year later. The patient was seen because she fell on the ice with complaints of pain at the base of her spine. X-rays show a forward displacement of the last two coccygeal segments.

May of the same year. The patient was having increased pain and marked tenderness and pressure over the lumbar sacral area at the left side and left sciatic notch: DX L4-5 intervertebral disc protrusion into the sciatic nerve. Medications: Tanderil and colbenamid.

She was treated with injections to the area and with medications through the following year when she started T.E.N.S. treatments. The electrodes were placed at L-S site and sciatic notch bilaterally, with good results.

After 1 week of T.E.N.S. therapy the patient was elated over relief obtained, and was able to move her left leg without pain. Proper utilization for home use of the instrument was demonstrated to the patient and her husband to insure proper placement of the electrodes.

She continues to have good relief of pain and has become more functional. She still continues on her medications of colbenamid and Naproxyn. The serum uric acid found to be elevated 3.8 mg - consequently colbenamid was continued.

CASE HISTORY 5: Diagnosis: Multiple Myeloma

Patient is a white female, age 58, who fell and broke her left hip 10 years ago. She had a prosthesis implanted.

An orthopaedic surgeon saw her with complaints of constant pain on the left hip with tenderness from L-3 to sacrum. She was treated conservatively with medication, brace and injections.

Over the next four years her pain increased over the greater trochanteric bursa and an excision of the bursa of the left hip was performed. The patient continued to have severe pain in the area, and an excision of scar on the left hip was performed with good results. She continued to do well for the next 2 years. At this time she was admitted again for consultation at which time various studies were performed and she was found to have a high gamma globulin content. An oncologist was called in consultation, who diagnosed multiple myeloma, placed her on proper medication along with Meprospan and Prednisone 5 mg.

The patient continued to have increasing pain in the low back area over the next 4 years, with pain on pressure at the left sciatic notch and over the left greater trochanter. She was started on T.E.N.S. therapy with two bars placed over the left trochanteric site. The first treatment was not successful (as often happens), but on the second, she found the pain to be less severe and was able to use the device at home. She was closely followed by telephone contact. After 6 months of self treatment, she reported she felt better, but her response to T.E.N.S. was decreasing due to increasing difficulties with pain in the left lower lumbar spine.

CASE HISTORY 6: Diagnosis: Carcinoma of the bladder

The patient was a white male, age 71, with a diagnosis of

bladder carcinoma, and collapse of the 4th lumbar vertebrae; osteoporosis.

He was first seen at home. His appearance and behavior was that of an acutely ill patient in extreme pain at right lumbar 4, and the right iliac crest. The patient appeared very weak and obviously had suffered a great weight loss. He refused to be hospitalized and was cared for by RN's on a 24 hour service. He used an electric heating pad constantly with obvious burn, but refused to discontinue to use it.

Medications: Demerol 75 mg q 4h for pain IM
Dilaudid 2 mg q 4h for pain IM
Phenergan 12.5 mg q 4h for pain IM
Norgesic q 4h
Valium 5 mg q 4h

T.E.N.S. was explained to the patient, his wife, and nurses. He was heavily medicated, therefore it was difficult to keep him awake during the procedure. The electrodes were placed at right lumbar 1 and 4, right iliac crest, and right posterior superior iliac creat.

Following the application of the electrodes, the patient was able to be without medication for 7½ hours.

The following day he was more lucid and apparently free of pain. The nurses regulated the instrument - Amp. 2, Rate 3, Width 2, Bal. 0. The nurse tried to assure the patient that T.E.N.S. would probably alleviate spasms.

The next day the patient ate lunch for the first time and apparently had no need for injections.

One week later the patient's condition deteriorated, and a pelvic scan revealed carcinoma of the bladder with no apparent metastisis.

He expired the following day.

As is demonstrated by the above cited case histories, T.E.N.S. is not the magic cure. What it does serve to do is reduce dependency on narcotics, and free individuals to return to a fuller life.

It is for this purpose that the Pain Center has been organized. This relieves the burden placed on primary care physicians, already frequently overworked, who are plagued with the "pain patient." At the center, we offer a potential solution to *some* of the problems confronting these patients and their physicians.

Careful records are kept recording the patient's responses to this form of therapy during the initial visits (Figures 4 & 5). A copy of the form is sent to the referring physician for his records, describing the dates of treatment, pain locations stimulated, and the results.

Pain is very personal, ofttimes debilitating, and always depressing — and sometimes misunderstood. Pain, to most, makes the responsibility of a home and occupation become an impossibility.

The staff of the pain center feels a great challenge when starting a series of T.E.N.S. treatments. In most instances, a great sense of satisfaction results. When the patient leaves the center with less or no pain, more freedom of movement, and possibility of becoming more functional and able to assume more physical responsibilities, then we feel T.E.N.S. has been effective. A close relationship develops between patient and staff. Frequent telephone contact is maintained, and follow-up evaluations on the patient's progress are made in the office every 3-4 weeks.

Pain Centers are being instituted in many large metropolitan areas. This method of dealing with human suffering seems to us most effective.

PATIENT____________________

ACCOUNT NUMBER____________

DIAGNOSIS__________________

____

____

<u>FIRST VISIT</u> DATE_______

AMPLITUDE_____RATE_____PULSE WIDTH-_____BALANCE_____

TIME PER TREATMENT____

COMMENTS____

____

____

SUCCEEDING VISIT 2 DATE____________________________________

AMPLITUDE_____RATE_____PULSE WIDTH_____BALANCE_____

TIME PER TREATMENT____

COMMENTS____

____

____

SUCCEEDING VISIT 3 DATE____________________________________

AMPLITUDE_____RATE_____PULSE WIDTH_____BALANCE_____

TIME PER TREATMENT____

COMMENTS____

____

____

Figure 4.

DATE: ______________________

NAME/ADDRESS OF REFERRING PHYSICIAN

RE: Patients Name ______________________________

Dear Dr.

Thank you for referring your patient, ______________, to the International Pain Control Center.

The patient received TNS treatments in this Center on the Following dates:

The Pain locations treated were

with TNS results.

It was recommended by the Registered Nurse treating your patient that he/she rent/purchase a machine, utilizing the unit at home for continued relief as instructed. The patient is to keep IPCC and you informed of his/her progress.

If we can be of further assistance to you, please do not hesitate to call; also feel welcome to visit our Center at any time.

Sincerely yours,

Figure 5.

Chapter 4

THE PHYSICAL THERAPIST'S ROLE IN PAIN MANAGEMENT WITH T.E.N.S.

GERALD N. LAMPE, R.P.T.

The physician is primarily responsible for the management of the PAIN PATIENT, but the ubiquitous nature of pain requires that the physician have paramedical personnel for adjunctive therapy for such cases. Physical Therapists work very closely with the physician toward the goal of providing the very best methods available for pain management.

Recently, the physician and physical therapist have been priviledged to witness and participate in an exciting and challenging surge in research directed toward answering the questions of what pain is, and how it is best treated.

Pain is still relatively undefined, and remains the most disabling symptom of the majority of diseases. However, progress has become very gratifying to the physician and therapist, but, most important of all, to the pain patient.

"We know you have pain. . . . .but you will just have to learn to live with it."

Gerald N. Lampe, Registered Physical Therapist, with offices in Kansas City, Missouri is a graduate of the Mayo Clinic School of Physical Therapy. Additionally, he is a diplomate of the Tao-Chi Acupuncture Society. He has written and lectured on Transcutaneous Electrical Neuro Stimulation.

This type of report to the patient has occurred too frequently. It may reflect a deficiency of the degree of comprehension or understanding of pain, and a basic inadequacy of the most recent traditional procedures available for the treatment of some types of pain. To everyone's benefit, this type of statement is being less frequently required as a diagnostic/prognostic report to a patient.

Transcutaneous *Electrical* Neuro Stimulation is the terminology we prefer to use. The more widely used Transcutaneous Neuro Stimulation could refer to heat, cold, or any other stimulus. T.E.N.S. specifically indicates the type of neurostimulation which takes place. An important characteristic of the contribution by T.E.N.S. is that this form of therapy is completely non-invasive and non addictive. Medication and neurosurgery, when they are effective in pain management, may result in significant adverse side-effects and/or irreversable invasion of the human body. If a non-invasive procedure, which in non-addictive and without significant side-effects of adverse nature can successfully control or abate pain, the advantages of that modality become obvious. In many cases, this is the alternative offered by T.E.N.S.

After one or more surgical approaches for analgesia, many patients face the report that, ". . . . .you must just learn to live with your pain."

Many clinicians have reported relief for patients in this category. They are not forced to endure their endless discomfort or suffering.

Because of intractable, chronic pain, many patients become legally and practically disabled, either because of the dysfunction induced by the pain, or the adverse side effects produced by the medications which are required to moderate the suffering. Previously disabled patients are again leading useful lives in their homes and at their occupations. For these patients, constant or periodic use of a T.E.N.S. device may abate their pain, or, at least moderate it to a tolerable level permitting an increased amount of activity. The industry responsible for product design and production has made great strides in manufacturing compact, portable, yet durable machines which can be worn by very active individuals.

Because of this asset, its use is not restricted to the level or type of activity which might impose limitations on one's occupation, recreation, or sphere of movement. The non-invasive nature of the T.E.N.S. current emitted makes it possible for a patient to wear and use a device 24 hours a day, if necessary.

That a patient can reject the dependency imposed by the pain, and that he can return to gainful employment, no longer hampered by suffering, are in themselves remarkable results. In many instances, the concurrrent decrease in medications required for pain control is as important. By reducing the amount of medication, the restriction of activity frequently imposed by drug side effects, is lessened or abated.

The T.E.N.S. course of pain management may be much less expensive. Most portable T.E.N.S. units cost approximately $400. It is not uncommon for a patient to spend $2,000 to $3,000 yearly for the medications required for analgesics to sustain pain relief.

In addition to reducing the cost of pain management through decreased medication, T.E.N.S. may significantly contribute to an overall cost decrease. Via the usage of T.E.N.S., it has been found that the average length of hospital stay for pain related treatment is frequently shortened. The decrease in the cost of hospitalization and related services may be substantial, simply from this point of view. A patient may continue this adjunctive therapy through self-administered treatments at home effectively and safely, after having been properly instructed by a professional.

Although T.E.N.S. is relatively new, third party payors and workman's compensation carriers will reimburse for evaluation and treatment with this modality, and for its rental or purchase.

Workman's compensation carriers tend to support the use of T.E.N.S. because of the possibility of the work injured patient returning to the job more quickly, thus cutting their liability for treatment and for compensation related to lost man-hours. Additionally, some workers who might not otherwise be able to return to work may be able to do so through constant or frequent use of the device.

Other third party payors likewise reimburse for the cost of equipment purchased, if a reasonable trial period indicates that this modality is beneficial to the patient.

Medicare, for example, frequently stipulates that a two week trial period be experienced and that a documented indication of this therapy's benefit be recorded before their intermediaries will reimburse for prolonged rentals or purchase. It is, therefore, beneficial to include a statement that a trial period has been undertaken with therapeutic results when writing a prescription for long-term rental or purchase of a T.E.N.S. unit.

WHAT IS T.E.N.S.*

It has been well established both by history and experience that such procedures as heat, massage, vibration, and itching are sometimes useful in modulating the symptom of pain. These procedures can, as a group, be categorized as pain modulators secondary to counter-irritation, which influences the interaction of the components of the sensory nervous system. The medical diathermies, hydro-collator packs, etc., historically utilized by physical therapists represent pain treatment with counterirritation. T.E.N.S. is also a form of treatment utilizing counterirritation secondary to the introduction of an electrical current to produce sensory modulation. Most T.E.N.S. units produce a direct current from a self-contained battery source, usually of an asymmetrical, biphasic wave form with a positive, rectangular wave component combined with a negative, inverted spike component, or a rectangular, monophasic wave form with only a positive component. The current frequently generated has a voltage range of 0-90 volts (60 m. amps.), and a rate range of 0-100 Hertz. The pulse width which is commonly a third adjustable parameter usually provides a pulse width duration range of 10-100 micro-seconds, in the monophasic wave forms, and 150-500 micro-seconds in the asymmetrical, biphasic wave form.

The phasic input provided by the T.E.N.S. device is thought to stimulate the large diameter afferent A fibers. According to the Gate Control Theory (Melzack and Wall, 1965), the stimulation of large diameter afferent A fibers relieves pain.

In my opinion and interpretation of the possible neuromechanisms for pain modulation based on this Gate Control Theory, the indication is that the stimulation parameters produced by most T.E.N.S. devices provide the electrical characteristics which should stimulate the large diameter afferent A fibers better than the smaller diameter C fibers, the stimulation of which would result in the perception of pain.

THE GATE CONTROL THEORY

This theory has been discussed in other Chapters 1,16. Its very name suggests that there is a gating mechanism in the nervous system. The location of this mechanism is in lamina II and III (substantia gelatinosa) of the dorsal horn. This Gate mechanism is an intermediate structure between the transmission cells of lamina V, which must be stimulated in order for a pain interpretation and response to occur AND the sensory fibers which, via the dorsal root, enter the dorsal horn at the surface of the zone of Lissauer and lamina I.

Restated, the T-cells must reach their threshold and be activated if pain is to be interpreted. The activity of the A and C fibers has the potential of eliciting a response of the T-cells. Before they can effect the T-cells, the potentials from both fiber types must pass through the substantia gelatinosa, i.e. the Gate. Whether or not pain results is determined by the relative activity in the large diameter A fibers and the small diameter C fibers. High levels of activity in the A fibers, by a negative feedback mechanism, "close" the Gate by "toning down" the effect of both large and small fiber input to the T-cells. Elevated activity levels in the C fibers "opens" the Gate, again by a negative feedback mechanism, which results in the net effect that input from both the large and small fibers reach the T-cells and create, by spatial or temporal summation, the excitation of the T-cells with perceived pain as the net result.

Often we see the clinical sympton of pain accompanied by a history indicating the occurrence of some noxious stimulus of an intense or prolonged nature. This type of pain is typified by musculo-skeletal injuries, cuts, burns, herniated disc syndromes, etc. These stimuli are medicated by the C fibers which have the net effect of facilitating tramsmission across the substantia gelatinosa, resulting in activation of the T-cells in lamina V, yielding pain.

This illustrates pain resulting in C fiber dominance over A

fiber secondary to excessive stimulation of C fibers. Some pain syndromes seen clinically illustrate pain resulting from a different type of neurological interaction. In some neurological pathologies, such as neuralgias, there is myelin sheath destruction and A fiber destruction, resulting in a decreased functional capacity of the A fibers. Although in this instance C fiber activity may be unchanged, the C fibers may become dominant over the A fibers, secondary to the decreased functional ability of the latter fiber group. Thus, the normal "balanced" A-C fiber interaction is altered by the A fibers becoming "submissive" to the C fibers.

THE CLINICAL SIGNIFICANCE OF THE GATE CONTROL THEORY

The Gating mechanism, or substantia gelatinosa, is contained in the dorsal horn on either side of the spinal cord. The activity within the substantia gelatinosa on one side may significantly influence the activity of its counterpart on the contralateral side. Therefore, to obtain the maximal Gating activity at a given spinal segment level, it is my suggestion that bilateral placement is very useful. Even in instances of unilateral symptons, once the proper electrode placement has been established on the involved side, the same placement is repeated on the opposite side of the body.

Again, because commiseral fibers connect the substantia gelatinosa on each side, so that one influences the other, special consideration is indicated in treating the peripheral nerve diseases which result in a differential loss of the larger afferent fibers.

In post herpetic neuralgia, for example, the skin may have an increased threshold for detecting touch stimuli and yet it may become hyperpathetic.

The first tendency, if T.E.N.S. is a selected modality, is to place the electrodes in the dermatome at which locus the patient reports the symptom of pain. In my opinion, although placement in this manner is not contraindicated, T.E.N.S. should be used in this fashion with caution. The differential loss of the A fibers will diminish the responsiveness to T.E.N.S.

when applied to the involved area, so the efficacy of treatment would be altered proportionately. The effectiveness of T.E.N.S. application, in these instances, will be enhanced by placing the electrodes in the contralateral dermatome of complaint. Utilizing the "normal" A fiber response in the contralateral dermatome will influence the substantia gelatinosa of the uninvolved side, which will, in turn, postively influence the substantia gelatinosa on the involved side. Improvement in pain modulation results when compared with placement only in the dermatome of the involved side.

The Gate Control Theory's basis appears to indicate that sensory input may influence the perception of pain. It would appear that using the T.E.N.S. for relief in patients where there is a marked sensory loss would render a decreased beneficial effect proportionate to the degree of sensory loss. Where sensation is lost in one extremity in which there is a complaint of pain, it is suggested that bilateral treatment will improve results.

Intense, well localized pain occurring with a contusion enters into a discussion of the Gate Control Theory, as does the duller, more diffuse pain persisting long after the initial trauma.

This theory may additionally offer valuable insight into the treatment of amputees, cervical and lumbar pain syndromes, and the beneficial results frequently obtained with articular facet mobilization, along with other noted clinical phenomena, discussed in other chapters.

APPROACH TO THE PATIENT

Because of the potential anxiety people may experience when anticipating "electrical" stimulation, because of the connotations of the word "electrical," we suggest that the initial contact with the patient should reflect the use of the word "Neuromodulation." Once the patient has experienced the neuromodulation current, an additional explanation of its electrical properties may be indicated.

It is beneficial to emphasize to the patient that one may terminate the treatment at any time to reduce the possible anxiety which may have been created.

Extreme caution should be maintained to avoid overt suggestion that T.E.N.S. will relieve the pain symptoms, in order to facilitate obtaining an objective assessment.

If feasible, the patient, with the cooperation of the physician, should discontinue analgesic medications six hours prior to T.E.N.S. treatment. This makes patient evaluation and the efficacy of T.E.N.S. in this situation more valid.

When following the routine course of taking the patient's history and performing the clinical evaluation, in conjunction with the data submitted by the referring physician, special characteristics of the pain symptom reported by the patient should be recorded accurately, and whenever possible, the clinician should map out the patient's area of pain.

ELECTRODE PLACEMENT

The efficacy of T.E.N.S. treatment depends greatly on the proper selection and placement of electrodes to ensure the most efficient modulation of the peripheral and central nervous system. The basis for proper electrode placement appears to rest in the proper evaluation of the dermatome/s in which the pain exists, so that trigger points within the involved dermatome/s can be coupled with the corresponding spinal cord segment level/s to influence the nervous system most effectively (Figures 1, 2, 3).

Random electrode placement has produced random results. It is important to emphasize that each professional who uses T.E.N.S. should duplicate or create a consistant, logical procedure for selecting electrode placement sites.

EVALUATION OF THE EFFICACY OF T.E.N.S.

Subjective reportage by the patient will be the prime source for evaluation of efficacy. It is useful to try to apply some objectivity to the patient's subjective responses by having him relate to the increments of a ruler. We utilize this "measuring device" to assess the patient's response before, during, and after treatment. To have some rating standard as a gauge to determine significant benefit, it is suggested that a 50% improvement, or better, reported to the physician or therapist, is required to constitute a positive response.

THE QUALITY AND INTENSITY OF CHANGE

When a patient reports the disappearance of pain, another sensation does not appear as a substitute entity. The response to T.E.N.S. treatments may indicate no change in the symptoms, a partial loss of pain, or a total abatement of it. At times, what may have initially seemed a failure is, indeed, a relative success, when the patient notes that the level of pain without stimulation is greater than during stimulation.

Once a positive response is obtained with T.E.N.S., this effect generally can be maintained for the duration of the utilization of stimulation. Frequently, it is observed that a beneficial effect is prolonged beyond the stimulation period.

Most frequently, the effects of T.E.N.S. are experienced locally, but changes may be noted in remote areas as well.

EFFECTIVE TIME OF ONSET, AFTER EFFECTS, AND EFFECTIVE GAIN

While pain relief during the period of stimulation is a useful parameter in assessing the response of the patient to the modality, other observations are also useful.

We consider the effective time of onset, defined as the amount of time required for pain relief to occur after the stimulating device is turned on. In general, this occurs within one-half to one hour, but may take place within a few minutes, or up to seven or eight hours. Frequently an accurate indication of alteration of the pain level may be noted by the patient after a 15 minute period.

The after effect, or time consumed by the interval from the termination of stimulation to the recurrence of pain, may be considered as the duration of relief.

The effective gain is measured by observing the decrease in the effective time of onset and increase of the after effect over a period of repeated treatments.

It has been my observation that the effective time of onset is inversely proportionate to the rate used in stimulation.

To hasten the onset of pain relief, it is suggested that rates of 75-100 c.p.s. be employed until onset of relief occurs. We have also found that the after effect is usually at least as long as the period during which pain suppression was maintained, and often is longer. The after effect appears more prolonged in response to stimulation at rates of 30 hertz or below. Therefore, once the onset of relief occurs in response to the high frequency utilized at the onset of stimulation, decreasing the rate for the duration of that treatment will enhance the after effect.

To determine a patient's progress from treatment to treatment, observation of the effective gain is useful. This is done via a comparison of the effective time of onset and the after effect with successive treatments. To accomplish this, the patient may be instructed to turn the stimulator on and record the interval which occurs until the pain is gone. The patient then turns off the stimulator and records the length of the interval until the pain reappears. As stimulation is repeated, both the pain suppression effect and after effect usually are enhanced. Through this technique, we aim to control the patient's pain through periodic applications, rather than by means of constant, prolonged stimulation.

SUMMARY

Clinical experience has permitted the observation that many chronic pain patients have significantly benefited from T.E.N.S. as an adjunctive therapy or, in some instances, as a primary therapy for treating pain symptoms. T.E.N.S. has given more complete pain modulation when compared with oral medications previously used.

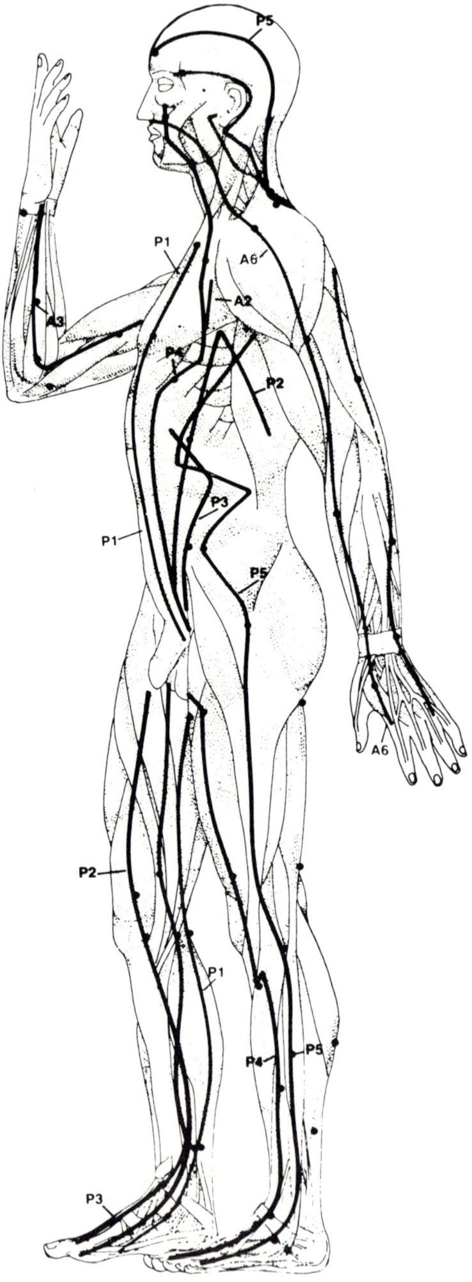

Figure 1. Suggested electrode placement for some of the most common pain problems. Provided by Med. General, Minneapolis, Minn.

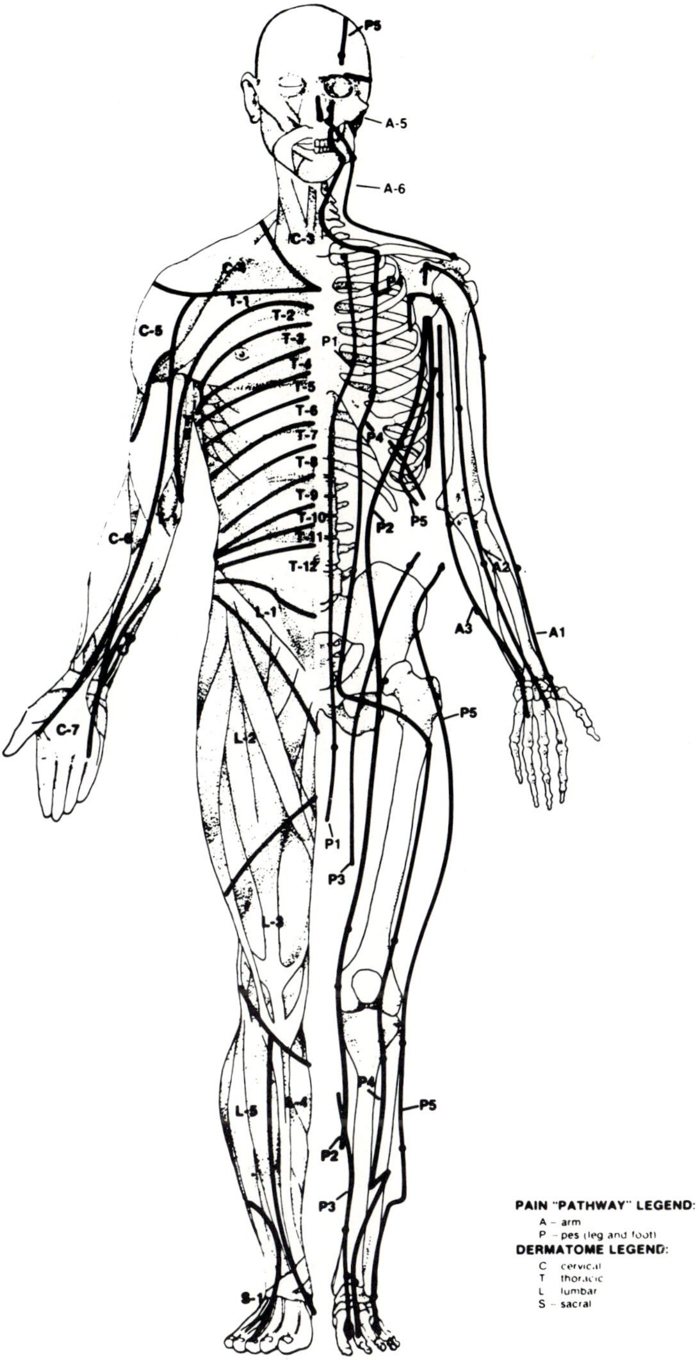
P5
A-5
A-6
C-3
T-1
T-2
T-3
T-4
T-5
T-6
T-7
T-8
T-9
T-10
T-11
T-12
C-5
P1
P4
P2
P5
C-6
A2
A3
A1
L-1
P5
C-7
L-2
P1
P3
L-3
P4
P5
L-5
P2
P3
S-1
PAIN "PATHWAY" LEGEND:
A – arm
P – pes (leg and foot)
DERMATOME LEGEND:
C – cervical
T – thoracic
L – lumbar
S – sacral

Figure 2

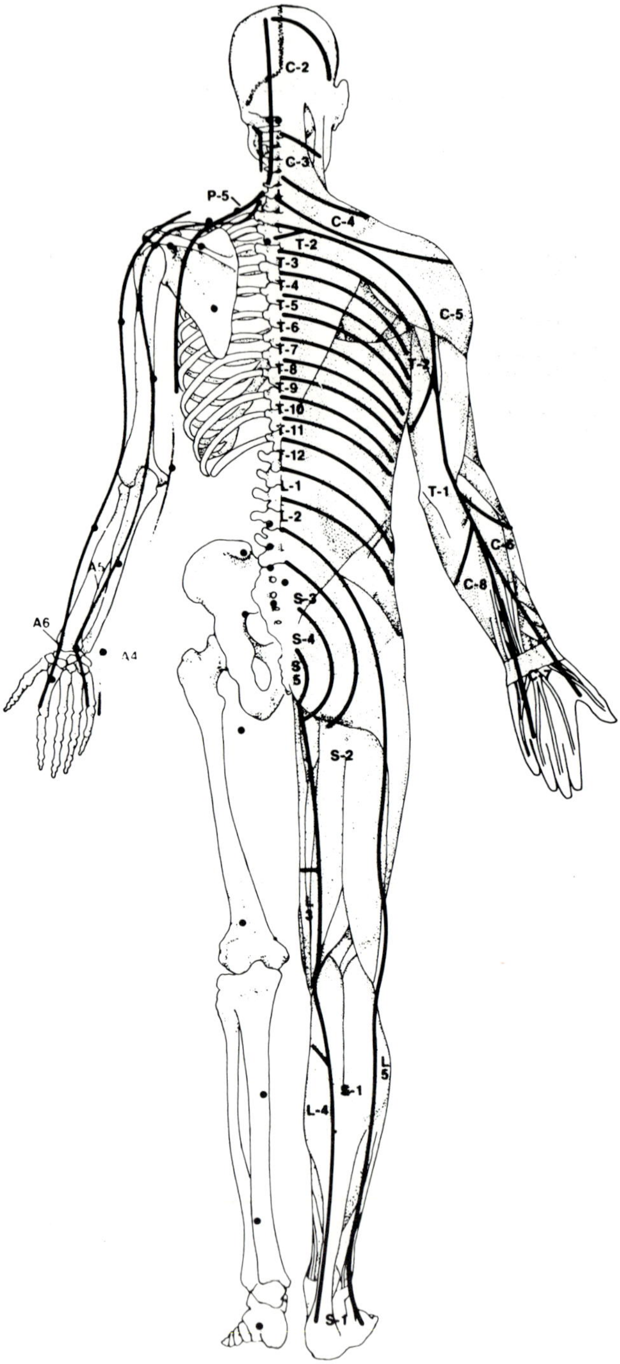
C-2
C-3
P-5
C-4
T-2
T-3
T-4
T-5
T-6
T-7
T-8
T-9
T-10
T-11
T-12
L-1
L-2
C-5
T-1
C-6
C-8
A6
A4
S-3
S-4
S
5
S-2
L
3
L
5
S-1
L-4
S-1

Figure 3

We have also noted that many patients, previously unsuccessfully treated by surgical intervention, received substantial relief from their symptoms with T.E.N.S. therapy.

Because of these very gratifying results in managing chronic pain, there is a tendency to overlook its utilization in the management of acute pain, post-surgical pain, or the suffering resulting from a terminal disease. Often acute pain responds more quickly than some chronic pain symptoms.

It is noted, in this book, in the Chapters by Hymes, Van der Ark, and others that post-surgical utilization of T.E.N.S. has been of great value. When this device is used in the management of postoperative pain, atelectasis and ileus, its value in these acute pain states has been demonstrated.

The suffering of terminal illness is sometimes eased by decreasing the accompanying pain with T.E.N.S. treatment, without the hypnotic effect of many analgesic medications.

My clinical experience, as a Registered Physical Therapist, has lead me to conclude that whether or not the Gate Control Theory is totally accurate in its explanations for the actions of T.E.N.S., the fact remains that this safe, non-invasive, non-addictive procedure for pain relief has been remarkably successful as an adjunctive treatment. It is a method which provided relief when other, more conventional pain management techniques had failed.

When a professional person provides a T.E.N.S. unit for long term use by a patient, the instructions for its use should include a precautionary statement that the T.E.N.S. DEVICE IS BEING PROVIDED ONLY TO THIS PATIENT FOR USE SOLELY IN CONJUNCTION WITH THE CONDITION FOR WHICH HE IS CURRENTLY BEING TREATED. SHOULD OTHER SYMPTOMS OF PAIN OCCUR AT A LATER TIME, THE PATIENT MUST CONSULT HIS PHYSICIAN BEFORE ATTEMPTING TO MASK THAT PAIN WITH THE T.E.N.S. UNIT. AT NO TIME SHOULD THE PATIENT PROVIDE HIS T.E.N.S. UNIT FOR USE BY ANOTHER PERSON UNLESS SPECIFICALLY PRESCRIBED BY THAT INDIVIDUAL'S PHYSICIAN.

Chapter 5

FROM DORSAL COLUMN IMPLANTS TO EXTERNAL TRANSCUTANEOUS NEUROSTIMULATOR DEVICES

Comparison and Appraisal of the Development of the Technique

C. NORMAN SHEALY, M.D.

With the presentation of Melzack and Wall's Gate Control of Pain Theory (1), it appeared obvious that we should be able to take advantage of the gate at some level.

Initially, and somewhat incorrectly, I assumed that we would have a better chance of controlling the gate if electrical stimulation were applied at the level of the dorsal column to the spinal cord, since activation of the beta fibers essential for inhibiting C fibers or pain activity might be expected to be accomplished more easily in the dorsal column, the only place in the entire nervous system where there is a physical separation of the various nerve fibers. Of course, this theory did not take into account the fact that electrical stimulation itself serves to differentiate between the fibers, since, fortunately, the threshold for activation of beta fibers is lower than that for C fibers.

Based on our original concept, our research proceeded with the experimental, and later, the clinical application of dorsal column stimulation. Between 1967 and 1973 we implanted dorsal column stimulators in a group of eighty patients. A huge variety of complications were experienced (Table 1). And, over the next few years, our results in terms of satisfactory results did not meet with our desires.

TABLE 1
DORSAL COLUMN STIMULATION
COMPLICATIONS

Type of Complication	*Frequency of Occurrence*
CSF leak	16
Electrode removed	5
Prolonged pain associated with operative wounds	10
Poor localization, inadequate stimulation	12
Hematoma, incisional (minor)	5
Uncomfortable paresthesia	7
Mechanical problems, requiring re-operation, re-positioning, or repair of wire	15
Partial paraplegia	3
Infection	1
Seroma	3
Total number of patients with complications	48
Total number of complications	77

Since one is dealing with a very subjective test, a "pain profile" was devised for use in assisting us with the determination of efficacy of treatment (Table 2).

With this technique to assess Dorsal Column Stimulation results, we consider as excellent those patients who have pain no more than 25% of the time, with a maximum of 30% intensity. We also consider as fair those who have pain 50% of the time, with a maximum intensity of 50%. In our initial six-month follow-up, we found excellent results in 20 patients, fair results in 31, and failures in 29.

With the same criteria in follow-up periods up to five years, and including a minimum of one year, we found excellent pain relief in only twelve patients, or 15%, fair pain relief in twenty-five patients, or 31%, and failures in forty-three, or 54% of the eighty patients operated. Fourteen of these forty-three failures occurred quite late, i.e., after at least three years. Good evidence suggested that the longer we investigated, the greater amount of failure would be found, resulting from such causes as breakage of wires after a prolonged time, etc.

Assessing the reasons for failure, we may state with reasonable certainty that twenty-four of the failure patients, or 30%, failed because of poor selection on the basis of personality, sometimes coupled with poor electrodes. Two of the failures were on the basis of electrode type, and three were from unknown reasons. Patients classified as poor personality choices

TABLE 2
PAIN PROFILE

On the columns below, grade yourself (circle) on these factors:

a. Your average severity of pain (100 = intolerable, excruciating, horrible);

b. Your average physical activity (100 = fully normal or as much as would be possible with *no* pain);

c. The average percent of time pain is felt;

d. Effect of your illness on your mood or personality (100 = totally withdrawn, panicked, overwhelmingly depressed);

e. Drugs consumed (M.D. will do ths).

a	b	c	d	e
Average Pain	*Average Physical Activity*	*Percentage of Time Pain is Felt*	*Effect on Mood*	*Average Drug Consumption*
0	100	0	0	0
5	95	5	5	5
10	90	10	10	10
15	85	15	15	15
20	80	20	20	20
25	75	25	25	25
30	70	30	30	30
35	65	35	35	35
40	60	40	40	40
45	55	45	45	45
50	50	50	50	50
55	45	55	55	55
60	40	60	60	60
65	35	65	65	65
70	30	70	70	70
75	25	75	75	75
80	20	80	80	80
85	15	85	85	85
90	10	90	90	90
95	5	95	95	95
100	0	100	100	100

were those whose MMPI's showed more than two standard deviations above the mean on four or more personality traits. In addition to these deviations, or at times without them, they were considered seriously disturbed by the surgeon prior to the operation. In the fourteen late failures, six of the patients had unresolved major personality conflicts; four were the outcome of gradual fading of stimulation; four are of uncertain cause. Late electrode problems, breakage in the wires or arachnoidal

TABLE 3
COMPARISON OF RESULTS (80 CASES) AND ELECTRODE TYPE

Three-plate Bipolar Electrode	(Tripolar; shielded bipolar)
Total implanted	34
excellent pain relief	9
fair pain relief	9
failure (5 late)	17
electrical wire break (after 3 years)	1

Three of the failures were due to mechanical pressure on the cord, i.e., paraparesis; three are of uncertain cause; the remainder were patients with serious personality problems.

Monopolar Tinsel Wire Electrode	
Total implanted	38
excellent pain relief	1
fair pain relief	12
failures (4 late)	24
electrical wire break (1 year or less)	4

This is an unacceptable electrode.

Bipolar Tinsel Wire Electrode	
Total implanted	19
excellent pain relief	2
fair pain relief	5
failures (5 late)	12
electrical wire break (1 year or less)	3

This is an unacceptable electrode.

Monopolar Plate Electrode	
Total implanted	2
excellent pain relief	1
failure (after five years)	1

Avery Bipolar Electrode	
Total implanted	1
Failure	1

Another major factor in success and failure is electrode position (107 electrodes)

	Excellent	*Fair*	*Failure*
Epidural	2	2	2
Endodural (interdural)	1	4	8
Subdural (extra-arachnoid)	12	36	40

thickening beneath the electrons probably resulted in many of the fading and uncertain cases.

While the patient's personality is of major concern, and contributory to success or failure, the type of electrode is equally important. In twenty-seven, or 34% of the patients, two electrodes were implanted to allow comparison with various positions of electrode or design. Comparing the results of the electrode types, we see that the three-place bipolar electrode is considerably more satisfactory than anything else tried in our patient series (Table 3).

There are two iatrogenic neurologic deficits which also have played major roles in our failure statistics:

	Excellent	*Fair*	*Failure*
Cingulumotomy	0	0	4
Cordotomy	1	3	8

No cingulumotomy patient has ever benefited, in our experience, with dorsal column stimulation or *any other therapeutic modality tried*!

Since 1974, technology is beginning to catch up with our original concept expressed in 1966, of allowing the insertion of the electrodes percutaneously. Although I have no personal experience with this technique, I am told that only 50% of the patients tested with the percutaneous device achieve adequate pain relief initially, and only 50% of those implanted achieve pain relief over a longer period of time. Late failures from wire breakage will be at least as common in this technique as with the implanted devices, but the morbidity should be considerably improved.

By the time we had done our first two dorsal column stimulation implants, it had become obvious that the patients had to be tested with external electrical stimulation prior to implants, initially to show them what the sensation was going to do to them. As soon as we began using external electrical stimulators, we found that a number of patients were getting adequate pain relief with this surface stimulation. This decreased the necessity of proceeding with implantation. Since that time, we have found external electrical stimulation to be considerably more efficacious than dorsal column stimulation. It is, of course, considerably safer.

At first we used laboratory stimulators through saline soaked sponges. A few months later, by early 1968, we were treating patients with Electreat, a battery powered external stimulator, which had been available on the open market since 1918.

Investigation of all standard wave forms — square wave, saw tooth, spike biphasic, sine wave, etc.— studied during the next two years lead us to the decision that the spike and the square wave were the only two really useful transcutaneously. In the fall of 1971, both Stimtech and Medtronic began producing external electrical stimulators. StimTechs were the square wave, Medtronics were the spike. During the ensueing years, Medtronic converted to their moderate size, dark brown TENS—an epimini square wave device.

Since 1974, companies manufacturing external stimulators have increased geometrically. Unofficial estimates suggest that there are between thirty and fifty companies putting out such devices at the present time. Many of these have been tried at the Pain and Health Rehabilitation Center, LaCrosse, Wisconsin. Some have been found in our work to be more satisfactory than others. . .although individual preferences enters here, and new adaptations are being made regularly on many of the devices.

We have found virtually all stimulators useful for *certain* purposes. It is essential to note that some patients respond favorably only to one stimulator, while failing to achieve relief with any of the others.

With one of the stimulators frequently used at our center, most of the patients use the device only 3 to 12 minutes, from four to eight times daily. From the therapist's point of view, this device requires more time in application than any other, but the end result, when satisfactory, justifies the effort. Patients must experiment with a wide variety of locations or body sites, and try reversing positive and negative electrodes to determine maximum efficacy. The most remarkable aspect is that stimulation is applied up to threshold for sensation, then reduced to subliminal. It seems to act either to block pain or to balance the electrical resistance. Interestingly, the amount of current tolerated below sensation varies a great deal, and may either increase or decrease during stimulation. A large variety of electrode sizes and configurations is possible.

Chapter 6

THE TREATMENT OF POSTOPERATIVE PAIN WITH TRANSCUTANEOUS ELECTRICAL NEURO STIMULATION

GARY D. VANDER ARK, M.D.

INTRODUCTION

Because Transcutaneous Electrical Neuro Stimulation has become acceptable as a verified method for the control of chronic pain, it seems logical that acute pain may also be controlled by this modality. Physicians using transcutaneous stimulation for chronic pain patients were probably the first to apply this treatment modality to their own acute aches and pains. Anecdotal reports of transcutaneous stimulation for relief of pain associated with ankle sprains and minor burns brought to life the potential of transcutaneous stimulation in the treatment of acute pain.

The use of Transcutaneous Electrical Neuro Stimulation to control acute postoperative pain was first described by Hymes *et al.* (1) They reported a remarkable decrease in postoperative pain, atelectasis, ileus, and duration of intensive care in treating patients who had had chest or abdominal surgery. Their experience has stimulated others to use their treatment modality.

METHODS

Transcutaneous Electrical Neuro Stimulation may be applied in several different ways in the acute postoperative patient. Hymes *et al.* (1,2) have used continuous electrical stimulation. Other authors have only used the stimulator on an intermittent basis (3). Pain relief usually extends beyond the period of stimulation.

Maximal relief is almost invariably achieved when the stimulator is first applied. Decreasing effectiveness with time is occasionally noted.

The placements of electrodes does not seem to be crucial to the success of this form of treatment. Generally, the electrodes have been placed above and below the incision. Proximity to the incision is not of great importance which obviously is an advantage in avoiding wound contamination.

The configuration of electrodes is also not an important factor in relief of pain. Various shaped electrodes have been used with each patient having his or her own preference. Most patients, however, note similar results with all shapes and sizes of electrodes.

Patients must determine appropriate levels of stimulation for their particular needs. Usually the patient selects an output which produces a comfortable buzzing sensation.

RESULTS

Obviously, it is very difficult to isolate the placebo effect of electronic gadgetry. In the initial study reported by Hymes *et al.*(1), the control group consisted of patients undergoing similar operations during a period of time prior to the use of transcutaneous electrical stimulation. In a study reported in the *American Journal of Surgery,* one hundred (100) randomized postoperative patients were given stimulators, and in all cases electrodes were applied above and below their incisions (3). Some patients, however, were given stimulators in which no batteries were present and other patients were given functioning stimulators. Each group of patients were given similar instructions. In this latter series of patients, twenty-five percent (25%) had complete relief of pain and fifty-two percent (52%) reported only partial relief. In the original report of Hymes *et al.* (1), few patients noted complete relief of pain, but the majority reported a subjective reduction of sixty to eighty percent (60-80%).

TABLE 1
CORRELATION OF RESULTS WITH TYPE OF OPERATION

Type of Operation	*Total No. of Patients*	*Complete Success*	*Positive Partial Success*	*Negative Partial Success*	*Failure*
Control Group					
Thoracic procedure	1	0	0	0	1
Inguinal hernia repair	5	0	0	1	4
Cholecystectomy	7	0	0	1	6
Appendectomy	7	0	0	0	7
Hernia repair	6	0	0	2	4
Miscellaneous	13	0	1	2	10
Total	39	0	1	6	32
Experimental Group					
Thoracic procedure	6	2	1	1	2
Vagotomy and antrectomy	2	2	0	0	0
Inguinal hernia repair	7	3	2	2	0
Cholecystectomy	8	2	3	1	2
Appendectomy	10	3	2	4	1
Hernia repair	2	0	0	1	1
Miscellaneous	26	3	11	4	8
Total	61	15	19	13	14

Table I illustrates the results of transcutaneous electrical neuro stimulation in one (100) postoperative patients. Of thirty-nine (39) control patients, thirty-two (32), or eighty-three percent (83%) experienced no pain relief from the mock stimulator. Seven (7) patients did have some degree of relief from the sham stimulators. All but one of the patients, however, had no objective information (i.e., decrease in pain medication) to support their claim of some relief.

The efficacy of Transcutaneous Electrical Neuro Stimulation in alleviating postoperative pain does not seem to be dependent on the type of surgical procedure.

Without doubt, relief in some cases has a psychological basis. Those patients, however, who appear most suggestive and/or hysterical invariably prove to be poor candidates for effective use of Transcutaneous Electrical Neuro Stimulation.

ADDITIONAL BENEFITS OF TRANSCUTANEOUS NEURO ELECTRICAL STIMULATION

Trancutaneous Electrical Neuro Stimulation in postoperative patients has obvious advantages over alternative methods of pain control. It is nonaddictive and does not produce the characteristic sluggishness and sedation of narcotic analgesics. As a result, patients deep breathe, cough, and walk much better. This led to a dramatic reduction in postoperative atelectasis in the reports of Hymes *et al* (1,2).

A decrease in postoperative ileus has also been reported. The exact mechanism remains conjectural, but it has been postulated that Transcutaneous Electrical Neuro Stimulation causes a direct effect on the autonomic nervous system (1).

Patients with less pain, atelectasis, and ileus require less time in intensive care units.

When transcutaneous electrical neuro stimulation is used following thoracotomy, movements of the shoulder on the side of surgery is significantly improved. Early range of motion removes the necessity for prolonged postoperative physical therapy.

CONCLUSION

It certainly seems obvious that Transcutaneous Electrical Neuro Stimulation is a significant adjunct to the alleviation of acute postoperative pain. Although transcutaneous stimulation is not a panacea as the future analgesic, its role should be assessed critically and not denied.

BIBLIOGRAPHY

1. Hymes A.C., Raab D.E., Yonehiro E.G., Nelson, G.D., Printy A.L.: Electrical Surface Stimulation for Control of Acute Postoperative Pain and Prevention of Ileus. *Surg Forum,24*:447-9, 1973.
2. Hymes A.C., Yonehiro E.G., Raab D.E., Nelson G.D., Printy A.L.: Electrical Surface Stimulation for Treatment and Prevention of Ileus and Atelectasis. *Surg forum,26:*222-4, 1975.
3. VanderArk G.D., McGrath K.A.: Transcutaneous Electrical Stimulation in Treatment of Postoperative Pain. *Am J. Surg,130*:338-40, 1975.

Chapter 7

THE POSTOPERATIVE APPLICATION OF TRANSCUTANEOUS ELECTRICAL NEURO STIMULATION

ALAN C. HYMES, M.D.

The modern use of transcutaneous electrical nerve stimulation for pain control was re-established independently and collectively by Long (1) and Shealy (2). In 1970 and 1971, they were looking for a means to evaluate the effectiveness of dorsal column implantation. This evaluation was done by transcutaneous electrical nerve stimulation (T.E.N.S.). Many patients subjectively noted significant reduction of chronic pain from T.E.N.S. alone. As a result of these findings, both Long and Shealy established pain clinics using T.E.N.S. therapeutically for chronic pain.

It seemed logical to apply these electrodes in patients with acute pain such as one sees following surgical procedures. We then applied T.E.N.S. therapy to a 62-year-old man who had undergone a thoracotomy the previous day. Within 20 minutes of applying stimulation to the posterior aspect of his wound over his right shoulder, he subjectively reported the lack of sensation of any pain. He could raise his arm directly overhead and touch the opposite shoulder behind his neck with no pain. The subjective observations were most striking. It seemed that this phenomenon deserved to be studied in more detail. Our initial investigation lasted several months. Intermittent treatments and continuous treatments were given to patients who had undergone a variety of surgical procedures. An historical control group was used reviewing patients who had similar procedures by the same group of surgeons in our institution (3,4).

In comparing the group treated with the historical control, it appeared as though there was a significant reduction in post-operative complications of ileus and pulmonary complications of atelectasis.

A forward randomized clinical study was undertaken to test the validity of our initial observations.

METHODS

Patients were categorized according to the type of surgical procedure and then randomized into either a treated or a control group. All patients had electrodes placed in juxtaposition to the surgical wound 4-6 cm away from the incision on either side. Electrodes were then connected to a T.E.N.S. unit. The light was covered in all instances. The control patient had the batteries reversed. The nurse applying the apparatus knew the patients receiving T.E.N.S., but the attending nurses and physicians who made most of the evaluations were not aware of the group randomization.

The signal from the T.E.N.S. unit was a modified square wave of 350-400 microseconds in pulse width. This had a frequency of 100-150 cycles per second. There was a maximum amperage of about 60 milliamps, however, the output was controlled by the individual patients. It was rare for the amplitude to exceed 30 milliamps as the sensation from a greater current was sharp-biting and uncomfortable causing stimulation of the underlying muscle as well.

The size of each electrode was 2″x8″some thoracotomy patients, four electrodes were used with dual unit output. Early in our investigation we used aluminum foil electrodes with a great quantity of gel held on by surgical tape. In the latter two thirds of the study, a non-sterile Karaya gum electrode was formulated to be self-adhering and conducting, thus obviating the inconvenience of gel and tape and the associated complications

The gel electrodes after application rarely maintained a homogeneous electrical current density, thus resulting in minor skin irritations even to first degree burns from the electrical current. In addition, the adhesive tended to tear the skin in some patients. Overall, there was about 50% complication rate of minor skin irritations from gel and adhesives compared to about 12% with the Karaya gum formulation.

It was extremely important to remove all the surgical prep solution and soap in as much as electrical stimulation on the skin with this material present usually caused pruritis and skin irritations.

Between 1972 and 1976, 875 postoperative patients were treated with transcutaneous electrical nerve stimulation.

All of the evaluation was done by attending nurses and physicians who, according to the protocol, did not know which patients were being stimulated.

The following parameters were noted: 1) Postoperative complications of atelectasis and ileus. 2) Length of stay in the Intensive Care Unit and in the hospital. 3) Semi-quantitative analysis was made of ability to cough before and after stimulation and in comparison of the two groups. 4) The use of narcotics postoperatively was noted.

Atelectasis was defined as incomplete expansion of a segment or subsegment of pulmonary parenchyma. This clinical diagnosis was confirmed in all instances by x-ray.

Ileus was defined as the absence of bowel tones by auscultation and the presence of a nasogastric tube beyond the third postoperative day.

RESULTS

ABDOMINAL SURGERY: Figure 1 shows the overall results of abdominal surgical procedures. There were 163 patients in the control group and 179 in the treated group. The overall incidence of postoperative atelectasis was 18% in the control and 9% in the treated. In the control group the rate of postoperative ileus was 9% compared to 3% in the treated group. Both these differences were significant.

The abdominal procedures which were done include gastrectomy, cholecystectomy, colectomy, and surgery on the abdominal aorta. In addition, there were a group of patients who had bilateral nephrectomy and splenectomy prior to kidney transplantation.

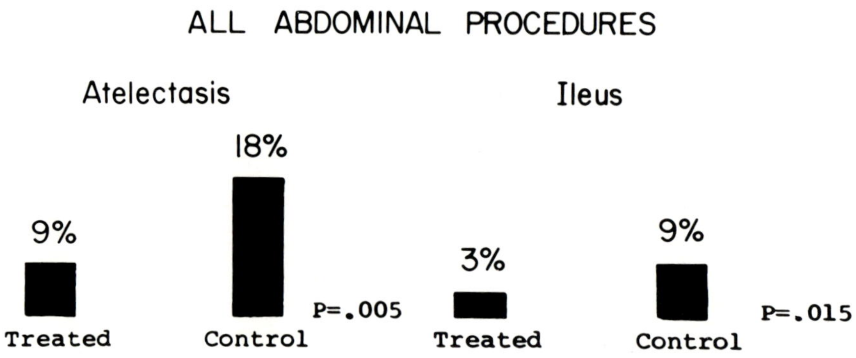

There was also a rather large group of patients who had miscellaneous procedures who were also treated. Because there was no control group, they were not included in this comparison study.

In general, the same trend followed in all subgroups with two notable exceptions. Patients undergoing colectomy and cholecystectomy showed no difference in postoperative complications between the two groups.

The patients who had undergone nephrectomy and splenectomy as a group complained that T.E.N.S. was a noxious stimulus, however, within ten to fifteen minutes most of these patients were sleeping following the initiation of T.E.N.S. therapy.

THORACOTOMY: In 42 patients who were treated with T.E.N.S., there was 14% incidence of postoperative atelectasis compared to 56% incidence in 43 patients in the control group. Qualitatively, the improvement in cough in the treated group was significantly better than the control group.

The angle of the humerus to the chest wall was measured on the first postoperative day following thoracotomy. Reduced pain enabled the treated patients to increase the angle significantly over the nontreated patients. In addition, there was a significant increment increase in the angle in the patients following the T.E.N.S. therapy. These results are noted in Figure 2.

Table I shows the results of patients who had postoperative ileus who were treated with T.E.N.S. The first group shows patients who were treated with medical management and

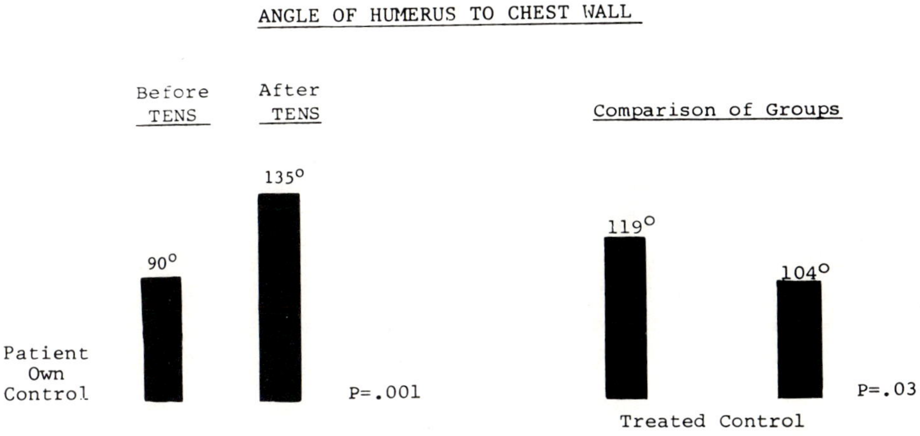

nasogastric decompression. The second group similar to the first, although patients did not have nasogastric tubes. The average postoperative day when T.E.N.S. was initiated was 5.5 days. As noted in the table, the majority of patients had flatus and bowel movements within 48 hours. There was still a small, but significant group of patients whose ileus continued beyond three days of electrical stimulation.

We made no attempt to control the narcotic usage. Somewhat to our surprise in our institution we found that the use of narcotics was related directly to the judgment of the attending nurses.

As a result, there were no demonstrable differences in frequency or total use of narcotics in any of our subgroups.

VanderArk and Mcgrath (5) specifically studied the use of narcotics in a very well controlled investigation. They found that T.E.N.S. provided good pain relief in 77% of the treated group as opposed to 17% of the control group. A similar study was done by Cooperman *et al.,* (4,6). They noted that 77% of their patients had good excellent results with 34% good excellent results in the placebo group. It is interesting that in both of these studies the placebo effect in the control groups parallels the results noted in drug analgesic studies.

Subjective reduction of pain in our experience was related to the following parameters: 1) The size of the electrodes. 2) The location of the electrodes. 3) The total electrical energy used.

The electrodes were each 2″x8″ and in many thoracotomy patients two pairs of electrodes were used with dual channel outputs.

The electrodes were placed 2″ to 4″ parallel to the incision. This area is over the maximum amount of trauma which, for the most part, is secondary to retraction. They were placed after a narrow surgical dressing had been applied.

To get the maximum amount of electrical current energy, a high frequency of 100-150 cycles per second was used with a pulse width of 350 to 450 microseconds. It was our opinion that the lower frequencies with reduced pulse width and, in particular, a spiked wave with a pulse width below 100 microseconds was not very penetrating and subjectively resulted in little or no pain reduction.

McCorkle (7) of Tempe, Arizona studied patients treated with T.E.N.S. following thoracotomy. He noted that very few of his patients experienced anything but mild discomfort following the surgery. He used two sets of electrodes with a stimulation area of 64 square inches with a dual output pulse generator. The signal was 450 microseconds with a rate of 150 cycles per second. The batteries were changed every four hours. I personally reviewed a number of his patients and with only one exception did any of them recall any postoperative pain. These findings as well as our own observations would lead to conclusion that the subjective reduction of pain as a result of T.E.N.S. is directly related to the area stimulated and to the total electrical energy put into these electrodes.

These independent observations are inconsistent with the "Gate Theory of Pain" as stated by Melzak and Wall (8), Campbell and Taub (9) noted pain and touch thresholds to a needle were significantly elevated following proximal nerve transcutaneous electrical nerve stimulation. They concluded that the analgesic effect from T.E.N.S. resulted from peripheral blockade of the A-delta fibers. In an independent study, Ignelzi and Nyquist (10) observed that T.E.N.S. alters conduction velocity in amplitude of the A-alpha, beta and delta waves with the A-delta (pain conduction) component showing the greatest reduction.

This conclusion does not imply that there is no central nervous system phenomenon. Many of the patients felt drowsy and, indeed, in one group as stated, most of the patients fell asleep following the onset of stimulation. These subjective observations are consistent with the known release of endorphins and/or enkephalins from direct electrical stimulation of brain structures (11). The extrapolation of these findings suggests the hypothesis that these polypeptides may be released by T.E.N.S. as well as other humeral agents such as serotonin (12).

Since our first reports, many manufacturers of T.E.N.S. units have promoted the use of this modality postoperatively. The most common electrode is a sponge gel surrounded by adhesive. In my opinion, all of these present electrodes are inadequate in size, except for very small incisions. Further, skin irritations from the non-homogeneous current densities and the adhesive make most of them undesirable. One electrode is a dry silver impregnated adhesive which also, in my opinion, is inadequate in size and is lacking homogeneous current densities.

Some manufacturers have promoted a spiked wave with essentially no pulse width whose power source can last several days. I have had no personal experience with these units, however, as stated it was our impression that low frequencies and/or narrowed pulse width did not subjectively reduce pain as well as the greater frequency with higher pulse width.

I personally disavow the references these manufacturers have made to our studies. These other systems need to be studied in a similar manner in order to claim efficacy and equivalency to the therapeutic value of T.E.N.S. as we had noted in our studies.

In summary, the overall conclusions are as follows:

1. T.E.N.S. using the parameters and electrode system as stated, reduces pulmonary complications by allowing patients to breathe deeply and to cough more effectively.
2. This modality is a noninvasive method in the prevention and treatment of ileus. The mechanism by which this occurs is not clear, although there is some indication that sympathetic tone may be inhibited.
3. There appears to be a subjective reduction in postoperative pain. This appears to be directly related to the surface area stimulated, the location of stimulation, and the electrical energy input into the electrodes.

TABLE I

POSTOPERATIVE ILEUS TREATED WITH TRANSCUTANEOUS ELECTRICAL NERVE STIMULATION (T.E.N.S.)

(Average day postoperative when T.E.N.S. started 5.5 days)

No. of Patients with N-G Suction	Day 1		Day 2	Day 3+
51 Patients	21 41%		16 31%	14 28%
N-G Tube Removed		72%		
	35 69%		5 10%	11 21%
Flatus		79%		
	25 49%		11 22%	15 29%
Bowel Movement		71%		
No. of Patients without N-G Suction				
42 Patients	31 74%		6 14%	5 12%
Flatus		88%		

Day 1 Day 2 Day 3+

31 5 6

74% 12% 14%

Bowel Movement 86%

0006

BIBLIOGRAPHY

1. Long, D.M.: Recent advances in the Management of Pain. *Minn. Med., 56:* 705, 1974.
2. Shealy, C.N.: Transcutaneous Electroanalgesia. *Surg. For., 23:* 419, 1973.
3. Hymes, A.C., Yonehiro, E.G., Raab, D.E., Nelson, G.D., and Printy, A.L.: Electrical Surface Stimulation for Treatment and Prevention of Ileus and Atelectasis. *Surg. For., XXV:* 223, 1974.
4. Hymes, A.C., Yonehiro, E.G., Raab, D.E., Nelson, G.D., and Printy, A.L.: Acute Pain Control by Electrostimulation. A Preliminary Report. *Advances in Neurology, 4:* 761, 1974.
5. VanderArk, G., and McGrath, K.: Transcutaneous Electrical Stimulation in Treatment of Post-Operative Pain. *Am. J. Surg., 130:* 338, 1975.
6. Cooperman, A.M., Hall, B., Sadar, E., and Hardy Jr., R.: Use of Transcutaneous Electrical Stimulation in Control of Post-Operative Pain. *Surg. Form, SSVI:* 77, 1975.
7. McCorkle, Jr., C.E.: Personal Communication.
8. Melzak, R., and Wall, D.W.: Pain Mechanisms; A New Theory. *Science: 150:* 971, 1965.
9. Campbell, J., and Taub, A.: Local Analgesia from Percutaneous Electrical Stimulation. *Arch. Neurol., 28:* 347, 1973.
10. Ignelzi, R., and Nyquist, J.: Direct Effect of Electrical Stimulation on Peripheral Nerve EvokedActivity. Implications in Pain Relief. *J. Neurosurg., 45:* 159, 1976.
11. Hosobuchi, Y., Adams, J., and Linchitz, R.: Pain relief by electrical stimulation of the central gray matter in humans and its reversal by naloxone. *Science, 197:* 183, 1977.
12. Shealy, C.N., Kwako, J.L., and Hughes, S.: Effects of Transcranial Neuro-stimulation upon mood and serotonin production. A Preliminary Report. *Il dolore, 1:* 13, 1979.

Chapter 8

AN ADDITIONAL APPROACH TO THE HANDLING OF POSTOPERATIVE PAIN

GERALD D. SCHUSTER, M.D.

Another area for utilization of Transcutaneous Neuro Stimulation has been tried for pain modulation in the immediate post-operative patient.

Others have successfully used this modality in thoracic and abdominal and cosmetic surgery for the past several months (Figure 1) and have reported on it in other chapters in this book.

I have instituted a specific non-narcotic post operative routine on patients requiring *spinal* surgery. The results have been most gratifying in several areas.

First - in the Recovery Room, the patients have responded more quickly without their narcotic sedation and have been able to return to their rooms more rapidly, with minimal discomfort.

We have been able to get the patients ambulatory more rapidly, with less associated pain. Ileus has not occurred as a post-operative complication, and the patients have remained much more alert and cooperative throughout their hospital stay. Many of these patients have been so well controlled in the initial post operative period that we have continued to allow them to utilize the T.E.N.S. unit on a specific time schedule when they have been discharged from the hospital.

No complicating factors have been found from the use of the sterile electrodes applied at the end of the operative procedure.

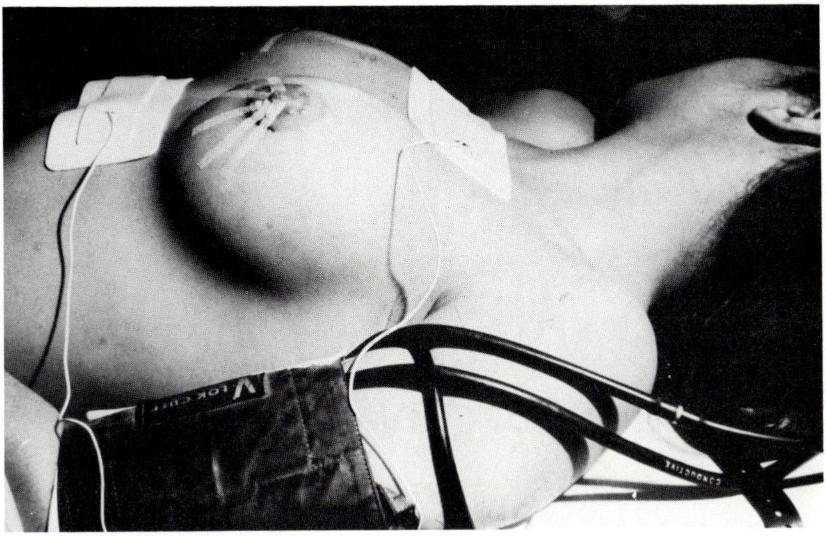

Figure 1 Ersek:
Post operative pain can be controlled with the use of commercially available pregelled adhesive foam electrodes. These electrodes are placed around the area of operative intent, in this case mammary augumentation, but remote from the actual incision.

The patients are instructed pre-operatively in the theory and use of T.E.N.S. The electrodes are removed and the system returned to the physician in about one week.

Each patient has been instructed on the use of the T.E.N.S. unit prior to the operative procedure, either by myself, or one of the center nurses.

The recovery room and floor nurses have also been carefully instructed on the use of the machine and skin and electrode care.

By the post operative day, the patients are able to control or modulate their pain themselves, and only need assistance with electrode replacement, or reapplying the gel once each 24 hours.

We are currently planning to expand the use of the device for surgical procedures involving the major joints of the body. It would be our hope that if pain can be better controlled without depressing the alertness of the patient through the use of narcotic agents, more rapid rehabilitation of operated joints could be obtained.

Chapter 9

POSTOPERATIVE TRANSCUTANEOUS ELECTRICAL STIMULATION AFTER APPENDECTOMIES

ROMAN KURZBAUER, M.D.

Adynamic or paralytic ileus is a very common complication following abdominal surgery.

After abdominal operations, the intestinal motility is impaired. The etiology of this condition is not yet clear.

Following appendectomies, there is also an ileus of transient character, normally lasting 24-48 hours, usually not more than 72 hours.

It is suggested that electrical stimulation, which is being investigated in the treatment of various diseases accompanied by chronic pain, could also work favorably in the postoperative period.

Neuromodulation in the management of postoperative complications should be achievable, for pain and ileus.

To verify these suggestions, an investigation has been carried out on patients who were operated upon for appendicitis.

The series was composed of 51 appendectomy cases who were treated with electrical stimulation, as compared with a control group of 50 similar patients.

All cases were operated on by the same surgeon and anesthetized by the same anesthesiologist.

There was an equal number of male and female cases. Mean age of both groups was 22.5 years, ranging from 15 to 35 years of age.

All were operated on under general combined endotracheal anesthesia. Time of operation was from 20 to 35 minutes. Any unusual or complicated cases were excluded from the trial.

During the postoperative period, the patients were administered analgesics - noraminopiryne - when required and intravenous fluids as necessary.

Intestinal peristalsis by ausculation was observed starting from the time of the completion of the operation until its appearance and after.

In the investigated group, 10 hours after the end of the operation, electrical stimulation was applied for the first time. This was performed by utilizing a stimulator that generated sine waves of low parameters with a frequency of 2-6 Hz. Two electrodes were located on both thighs - lateral aspect - and linked with the stimulator by a "Y" shaped wire. To close the circuit, another electrode was placed in the lumbar region.

Blood pressure and pulse were monitored throughout the session of stimulation, but no appreciable alterations were observed.

The time of each session was approximately 15 to 20 minutes.

Transcutaneous electrical neuro stimulation was then repeated twice, that is 5 and 10 hours after the initial session, or at the 15th and 20th post-operative hour.

RESULTS OF THE TREATMENT

In the control group, the average time of adynamic ileus until the reappearance of the peristalsis was approximately 26 hours. In the investigated and stimulated group, the effects are presented in three sets. In 33 cases, or 65% of the patients, peristalsis appeared following the initial session of electrical stimulation, between the 10th and 11th hour. The intestinal motility was rather weak during that period, and it lasted for abour 2-3 hours.

The seccnd session of electrical stimulation five hours later produced peristalsis in 46 patients, or 91% of all cases. This was strong enough so that the next, or third session was no longer necessary for these patients. In the remaining 5 patients, 9%, peristalsis appeared after the third and final session, i.e. 20 hours after the end of the operation.

Mean time of peristalsis reappearance in the stimulated group was 14 hours. That is 12 hours earlier than in the control group.

Postoperative pain was also observed and evaluated during the first few days after surgery.

Alleviation of pain, though not complete, was striking in the electrically stimulated group. Patients seldom required analgesics. Even if the relief from pain is only 50-80%, that is enough to enable the patients to move more easily in bed, thus avoiding any lung complications.

CONCLUSIONS

Electrical stimulation in the postoperative period for the prevention of various complications should become a strong and effective weapon in the hands of the surgeon.

Possibly, in major operations, many serious complications could be prevented by using this method even without additional drug therapy.

Electrical stimulation is very simple and safe to use, and no undesirable side effects were observed, nor are any to be anticipated in the future.

The mechanisms of the electrical stimulation as observed in the chronic pain control and in the postoperative management is not yet clear, but a sympathetic involvement and open mind to this new technique is recommended.

Transcutaneous Electrical Neuro Stimulation could become a routine method in the postoperative period in abdominal and thoracic surgery.

Chapter 10

ELECTRICAL STIMULATION OF VARICOSE ULCERS

ROMAN KURZBAUER, M.D.

Varicose ulcers are very common and still remain an unresolved therapeutic problem.

The number of patients with these ulcers is steadily increasing. The treatment is generally administered by surgeons or dermatologists. On the one hand, the surgeons are performing all kinds of reconstructive operations to cover the ulcers, while, on the other hand, the dermatologists are strictly adhering to the conservative method of treatment. Neither procedure is proving totally effective.

Electrical stimulation has been shown to be effective in many cases with chronic pain. It was intended to carry out a clinical trial to investigate and evaluate electrical stimulation for the pain relief and in the progress of healing of these troublesome varicose ulcers.

For the investigation, 61 patients with varicose ulcers were submitted to electrical stimulation therapy. There were 40 female and 21 male cases studied.

In the experiment, a stimulator working on the following parameters has been used:

Shape of current	-	sine wave
Frequency	-	approx. 2 Hz
Voltage	-	0 - 20 Volts
Intensity	-	200 - 300 microamperes

All of the patients were previously treated by all conventional methods for many months or years, some up to 15 years. They were all informed of the experiment, and full consent was obtained from all patients in the series.

During the therapy with electrical stimulation, no other drugs were administered, except dressings with rivanol. Analgesics were inititially reduced and then stopped altogether. Only fifteen in-patients were in the series. The remainder were out-patients, who reported as ordered for the session.

The electrodes were transcutaneous or needles applied below or above the knee, with the second electrode on the dorsum of the foot. Both electrodes were coupled with the stimulator by clips and wires. When needle electrodes were used, lower parameters as to voltage and intensity are utilized.

During the session of approximately 15 minutes duration, monitoring of pulse and blood pressure was maintained. The sessions were repeated as many times for a period of weeks. If there was evidence of improvement in healing of the ulcers, the treatment was continued until the final result was achieved.

All sessions were only performed in the supine position.

There were no undesirable side effects observed during the sessions, and throughout the treatment.

Results: The effects of the therapy were estimated according to:

1. Decrease or healing of the ulcer.
2. Relief or alleviation from pain due to ulcers.

Decrease of the size of the ulcers was obtained after a few weeks, i.e. 15 to 25 sessions, by approximately 50% reduction in the initial size. This was more evident in men.

Healing of the ulcers was observed in 31 patients after a period of approximately 3 months. In the follow-up, there were some relapses of ulcers, which were again treated in the same manner.

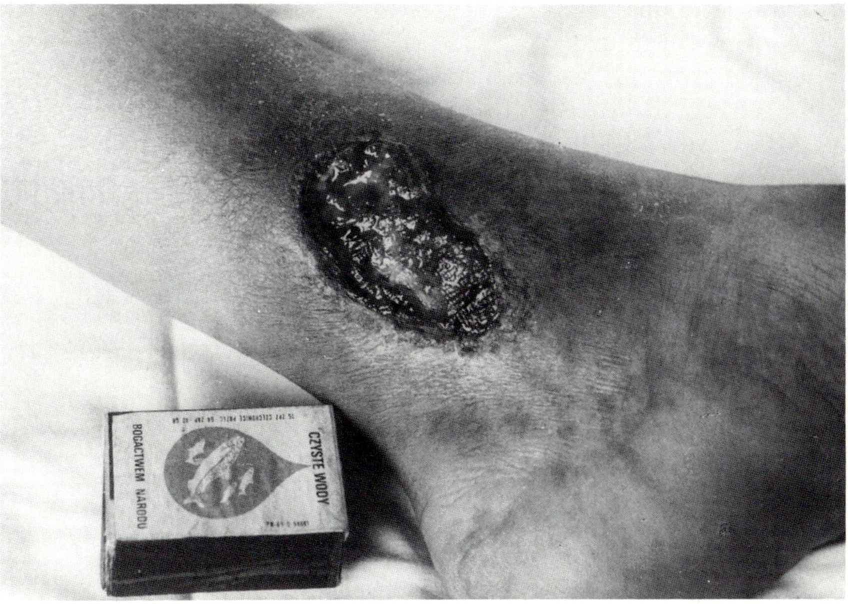
CZYSTE WODY
BOGACTWEM NARODU

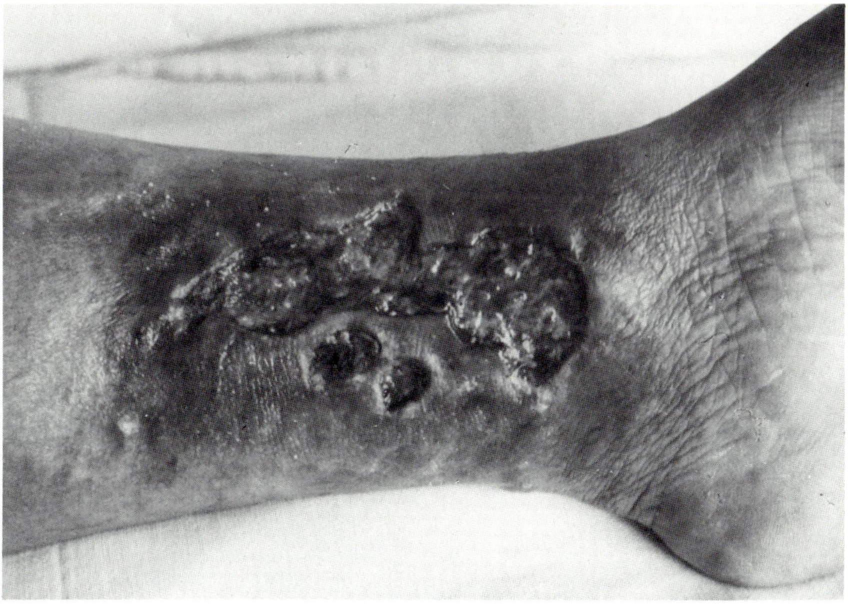

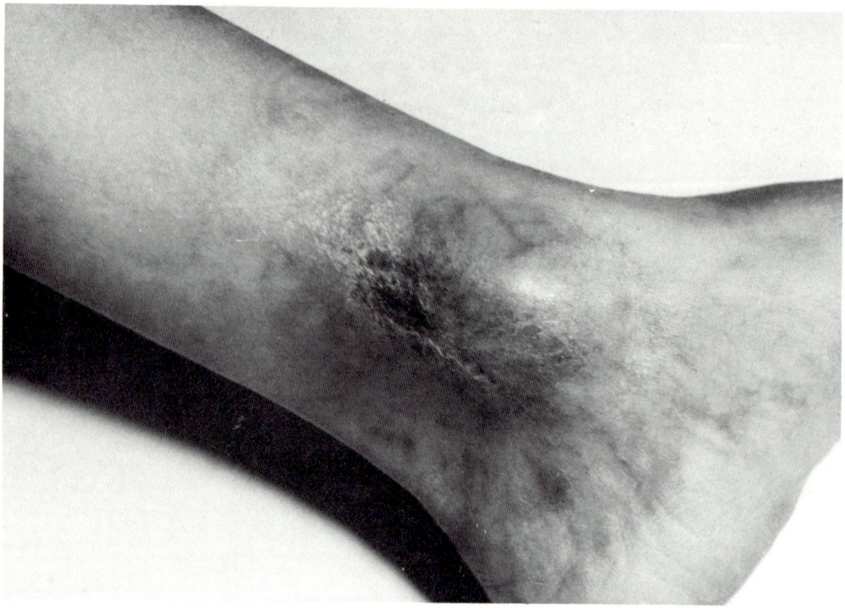

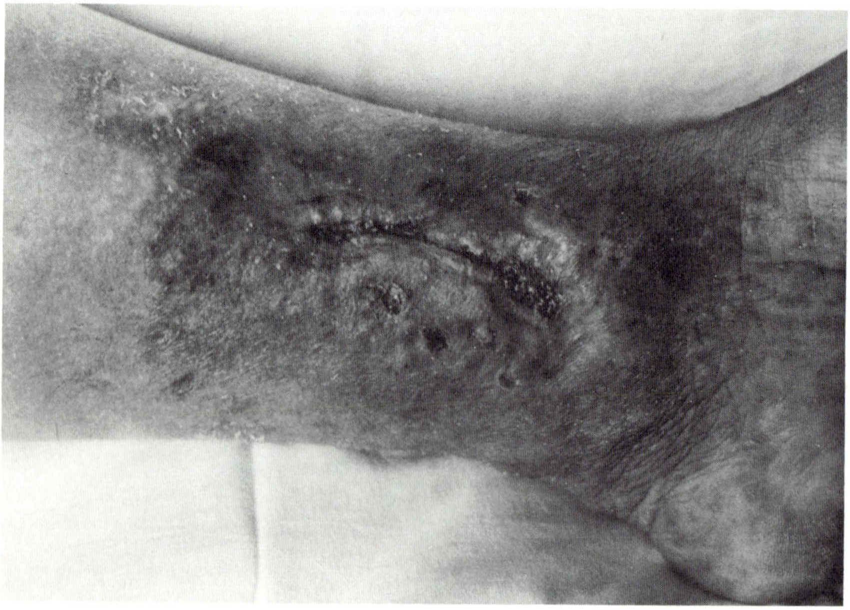

Illustrations A and B show ulcers prior to electrical stimulation, whereas A_1 and B_1 show the improvement in both cases.

A significant number of patients experienced alleviation of pain to the extent that they required no further analgesics. All patients in the series experienced alleviation of pain.

This form of treatment is especially recommended in patients with a long case history of ulceration problems. If not totally successful in its own right, electrical stimulation may be combined with other methods of therapy for control and alleviation of this troublesome condition.

Chapter 11

TRANSCUTANEOUS ELECTRICAL NEURO STIMULATION IN THE MANAGEMENT OF PAIN IN SPINAL CORD INJURED PATIENTS

ROSS DAVIS, M.D. & RICHARD LENTINI, M.S.

From the instant of spinal cord injury, with its loss of function, the individual experiences many deep and traumatic emotional reactions. The totality of the depths and extent of the injured person's feelings and thoughts are most difficult to appreciate. The reaction to the reality of being paralyzed is difficult enough to accept, but the reality of not recovering is perhaps the greatest single concept with which the patient has to deal. The resulting grievance over the loss of function is a paramount problem to overcome. The tincture of time is necessary and a period of mourning must pass for the individual to accept the devastation which has altered life's perspective for him. A usual pattern of emotions seen are those of depression, aggression, passivity, dependence, and certainly denial. A new start can be made in life by coping with his problems through rehabilitation and vocational training. This permits him to see himself as a person of worth.

Complicating the already paralyzed and devastated individual is the factor of pain. Essentially, pain arises at three different sites, and, of course, can be in combinations: at the site of trauma, pain referred from damaged roots, and pain experienced below the level of injury.

Transcutaneous Electrical Neuro Stimulation (TENS) plays a definite role in the conservative management of spinal cord injured patients with pain and suffering. However, its effectiveness has been found to vary depending upon which of the three types and sites of the pain are present and the psychological states of the patients (1).

PROCEDURES AND TECHNIQUES

In a study of 31 patients with spinal cord injury, the patients were tested with T.E.N.S. They ranged in age from 23 to 68 years and had lesions from C3-4 to L5. Many required analgesics such as pentazocine (Talwin), carbamazepine (Tegretol) and oxycodone (Perdodan) for relief. Five of the patients in this series had cordotomies, with subsequent return of pain.

T.E.N.S. stimulators manufactured by several companies were used. All of these devices are solid state, battery operated pulse generators that deliver variable electrical spike pulses to a pair or pairs of electrodes. The voltage amplitude and pulse rate were adjusted to suit the patient. When necessary, the pulse width was also adjusted. To minimize battery drain, the pulse rate and width controls were usually kept at the lowest setting agreeable to the patient.

We designed the electrodes used (2), since those supplied with the devices were, in many cases, not large enough to completely saturate the painful areas of most patients, with current. Also, except for the newer conductive rubber electrodes, those furnished were bulky and difficult to keep taped to the skin in a comfortable position. The patients made our own electrodes, utilizing ordinary hospital materials. (Fig. 1)

Our electrode is a much larger cutaneous electrode than those supplied by manufacturers with the stimulators. It covers more dermatomes, enabling it to stimulate larger areas and to alleviate pain where the small electrode has not worked. It is easily made from an aluminum foil strip held against the skin with adhesive tape. A bare wire goes between the aluminum and the adhesive tape. These electrodes are made as long as desirable, and in equal pairs (Fig. 1).

Three categories of treatment results were used, stemming from the amount of relief obtained from the stimulator. These included successes, partial successes and failures. Those cases which were considered successes were those in which the patient claimed enough relief to warrant wearing the TENS unit whenever the pain was present. At least a reduction in analgesic dosages were recorded. In the partial success category, the patients reported a slight amount of relief, but not enough to motivate them to set up the equipment, tape the electrodes on, and keep the device with them. The patients with failures claimed no relief at all.

Before any of the patients in the series were placed into any of the above categories, they were allowed to use the device for at least three days. Some of the patients were not evaluated until they had tried the device for more than one month. The time trial of a few days was felt necessary to eliminate patient bias about the device. For example, many of the patients had known of the device, were anticipating using it, and at first claimed relief; however, after several hours of use, they complained of the stimulation not being effective enough to warrant continued use.

SITE OF TRAUMA

Following trauma, there is tissue injury to areas such as the vertebral column, ligaments, muscles and tendons, connective tissue, and the nerves in these areas. Generally, this pain does not last more than a few weeks or even a month or two and does dimish with healing. However, if instability of the vertebral column persists, then with movement comes aggravation of the pain. Damaged facet joints may become arthritic and with the instability and movement, more discomfort is manifested. Fusion of the unstable spine generally stops this pain. Chronic, intractable pain at the site of injury, however, can be helped by the use of T.E.N.S. Eleven of the patients thus treated have had good relief from pain (3). Where facet arthritis is a problem, then the injection of steroids into these joints has been helpful. If relief is only somewhat temporary, then a facet rhizotomy can be performed with some good results (4,5).

PAIN FROM RADICULAR DAMAGE

With vertebral damage, such as fracture or extruding disk material, the nerve root(s) may be compressed or torn. Furthermore, as the months pass, the roots in the area of damage may become involved in a chronic process of adhesive arachnoiditis. Pain emanating from damaged roots is often described as sharp, shooting, aching, burning, tingling, and even cramping, as well as numbing. These discomforts radiate into the dermatomal areas supplied, which is the transitional zone between sensation and anesthesia. Often in this area there is a band of hyperesthesia.

In cervical, upper and mid-thoracic regions spinal cord injury affects one to four roots at the most, however, in the lower thoracic and lumbosacral area (cauda equina) many more roots become involved so that the area of pain is considerably greater, and consequently some patients have the most miserable pains spread through a wide area of the lower extremities and trunk. This may be such that the patients become debilitated and anorexic with a developed reliance on heavy narcotic analgesics.

The question of any extra-dural pressure on the roots should be settled early, if necessary by radiologic examination, including myelography. If there is a block encountered while attempting to inject the myelographic dye from below, it is advantageous to instill the dye via a lateral cervical (C2) puncture. If a torn disc or fractured laminae is found compressing the root(s), then a considerable amount of pain can be relieved with a possible return of function if either a decompression laminectomy or anterior discectomy with fusion is carried out depending on the circumstances. With laminectomy, torn roots, if few in number, can be dealt with by a section of the posterior root for pain relief (posterior rhizotomy).

Extensive and severe intractable pain resulting from radicular damage especially in the cauda equina area provides the most difficult management problem. Considerable effort should be expended for a thorough physical, psychological, and social evaluation before any treatments are instituted. It is of primary importance to determine the patient's psychological status — what are his emotional feelings, is he perhaps somaticizing his anxieties as pain. Is the patient using the pain as a means of communication to obtain his wishes or sidestep his obligations?

When evaluating cauda equina damage, it must be remembered that many of the nerve roots still have partial function and that an increase in pain or discomfort may indicate that the genitourinary, gastrointestinal, or skeletomuscular system could be involved in a pathological process. A search of the skin for breakdown or underlying developing pressure lesions should be undertaken, as well as evaluation for possible thrombophlebitis and latent fractures of the lower extremities, and possible myositis ossificans.

After all of the above factors are looked for, and the best treatment of the pathology carried out, then the patient should be placed on a well-regulated diet, with nursing, physical and occupational therapy programs. The application of Transcutaneous Electrical Neuro Stimulation was found to be beneficial in suppressing the pain in 8 of 16 cases (Table 1) where the conus and/or cauda equina was damaged (6,7). Carbamazetine (Tegretol, Geigy) or diphenylhydantoin (Dilantin, Parke-Davis) have been useful for many patients in reducing the burning type of radicular pain. It is stressed that pain medication should be given regularly instead of when necessary. In this way, there is less interaction between the patient, the pain and the nurse in regards to the significance of taking medication. In this way, the strength of medication may be decreased. Hopefully, through the psychologist and social worker with the aid of nursing and medical personnel, family and occupational adjustments can be corrected, as well as the overall emotional state of the patient. It cannot be stressed enough that in this type of program the management of the most severe, intractable pain problem may be greatly rewarding.

The use of dorsal column stimulator implantation in patients with spinal cord injury has not been helpful in the majority of cases. Cases collected from 9 different clinics in the United States with a total of 27 patients have shown successful pain suppression in about one-third of the cases.

We should keep in mind that this is a basically nondestructive procedure, and now, with the increasing developments in T.E.N.S. patients who may best benefit from implantation can be better selected. The conservative pain rehabilitation program outlined above should be undertaken primarily.

PAIN EXPERIENCED BELOW THE LEVEL OF INJURY (SPINAL CORD DYSESTHESIAS

Following the loss of normal feeling below the level of injury, the majority (82-94%) (8,9) of spinal cord injured patients described various feelings such as numbness, burning, tingling and dull aches. The intensity of these feelings gradually recede as the patients accept the new situation and become more active. Usually patients will not describe them unless asked. These sensations, when intense, have been termed phantom pain or central pain (10). Even the persistance of a sympathetic nerve pathway has been proposed as the mechanism (11,12).

It is known that these dysesthesias are influenced by various factors such as depression, anxiety, inclement weather, alcoholic excesses, as well as marijuana, cigarette smoking, exercise and fatigue. Poole (13) described two patients who developed severe burning sensation in the legs with smoking. Both patients had complete cord injuries and even after the excision of the intra-spinal scar, the burning pain provoked by smoking still persisted.

Kruger (14) studied a patient with a mid-thoracic lesion who had no awareness of his body below the nipples. However, after commencing to smoke, the patient would have a "waking up" sensation in his left leg and toes.

One of our patients who suffered a C5 complete spinal cord injury felt he had an extra pair of legs which at times were tied up in knots. However, following range of motion of the lower extremity, he did feel a relaxation and an untieing of the legs settling in a more relaxed position. Of 7 patients who had smoked marijuana and who had phantom pain (15), one described that smoking increased sensation while three found that it decreased, however, two were distracted or paid less attention to the pain, whereas one had no effect. From these findings little can be deducted as to the efficacy of marijuana, although it is noted that it does alter the perception of the phantom pain.

In some patients, new pathology developed below the level of injury may somehow accentuate the burning experienced. Usually there is a concurrent increase in the spasticity observed. The mechanism is unclear, although perhaps there are meager or high threshold sensory pathways that have survived or perhaps it is a function of the sympathetic nervous system (11,12).

Investigation and management of the patient with intractable, severe phantom dysesthesias are similar to that described for the radicular-type pain, including a thorough history and physical as well as laboratory investigation combined with an evaluation of the patient's psycho-social behavior. Carbamazetine (Tegratol, Geigy) or diphenylhydantoin (Dilantin, Parke Davis) have been useful in reducing the dyesthesias. Narcotic analgesics are not recommended as they are most habit forming. The use of Transcutaneous Electrical Neuro Stimulation in these cases has not been of significant success in suppressing pain in this group (Table 2) (6,7). Eleven patients were treated with T.E.N.S. but only two had some relief of their discomfort.

In this group surgical treatment is strongly contraindicated as failure has been the result (3).

SUMMARY

The results of Transcutaneous Electrical Neuro Stimulation in treating 31 patients with spinal cord injury have been presented. Success and failure are indicated as relative to injury location and the type of pain perceived. Results indicate that pain at the site of injury is treated more successfully than radiating or central pain.

BIBLIOGRAPHY

1. Davis, R.: Pain and suffering following spinal cord injury. *Clin. Orthop.,112*:76-80, 1975.
2. Lentini, R., Davis, R., Goldstein, J.: Modifiable inexpensive electrodes for transcutaneous stimulators. *J. Neurosurg.,41*:262-264, 1974.
3. Davis, L.: Treatment of spinal cord injuries. *Arch Surg.,69*:488, 1954.
4. Fox, J., Rizzoli, H.: Identification of radiologic coordinates for the posterior articular nerve of Luschka in the lumbar spine. *Surg. Neurol., 1*:6:343, 1973.
5. Shealy, C.N.: Percutaneous frequency denervation of spinal facets. *J. Neurosurg.,43*:488-451, 1975.

6. Davis, R., Lentini, R.: Transcutaneous nerve stimulation for treatment of pain in patients with spinal cord injury. *Surg. Neurol.*,*4*:100-101, 1975.
7. Lentini, R., Davis, R.: Proceedings of American Association Neurological Surgeons, Paper #60, Session VIII, April 24, 1974.
8. Heyl, H.: Some practical aspects in the rehabilitation of paraplegics. *J. Neurosurg.*,*13*:184, 1956.
9. Pollock, L.J., Brown, M., Boshes, B., Findelman, I., Chor, H., Arieff, A.J., and Finkle, J.: Pain below the level of injury of the spinal cord. *Arch. Neurol. Psychiat.*,*65*:319, 1951.
10. Holmes, G.: *Pain of Central Origin. Contributions to Medical and Biological Research.* New York, P.B. Hoeber, *1*:235, 1919.
11. Davis, L., Martin, J.: Studies upon spinal cord injuries II. The nature and treatment of pain. *J. Neurosurg.*,*4*:483, 1947.
12. Freeman, L., Heimburger, R.: Surgical relief of pain in paraplegic patients. *Arch. Surg.*,*55*:433, 1947.
13. Poole, J.: Conference on spinal cord injuries. Army Service Forces: Second Command Hospital. Thomas M. England General Hospital, Atlantic City, N.J. October 20, 1945; p. 149.
14. Krueger, E.: Management of painful states in injuries of the spinal cord and cauda equina. *Am. J. Physiol. Med.*,*39*:103, 1960.
15. Dunn, M., Davis, R.: Perceived effects of marijuana on spinal cord injured males. *Paraplegia*,*12*:175, 1974.

TABLE 1
RESULTS OF TRANSCUTANEOUS NERVE STIMULATION
ACCORDING TO SITE OF LESION

Site of Lesion	*No. of Cases*	*Successes*	*Partial Successes*	*Failures*
cervical	4			4
thoracic	11	5		6
conus, cauda equina	16	6	2	8
Total	31	11	2	18

TABLE 2
RESULTS OF TRANSCUTANEOUS NERVE STIMULATION
ACCORDING TO SITE OF INJURY, RADICULAR OR CENTRAL PAIN

Type of Pain	*No. of Cases*	*Successes*	*Partial Successes*	*Failures*
at site of injury	4	3		1
at site of injury, radicular	6	3	1	2
at site of injury, central	1	1		
radicular	9	2	1	6
central	11	2		9
Total	31	11	2	18

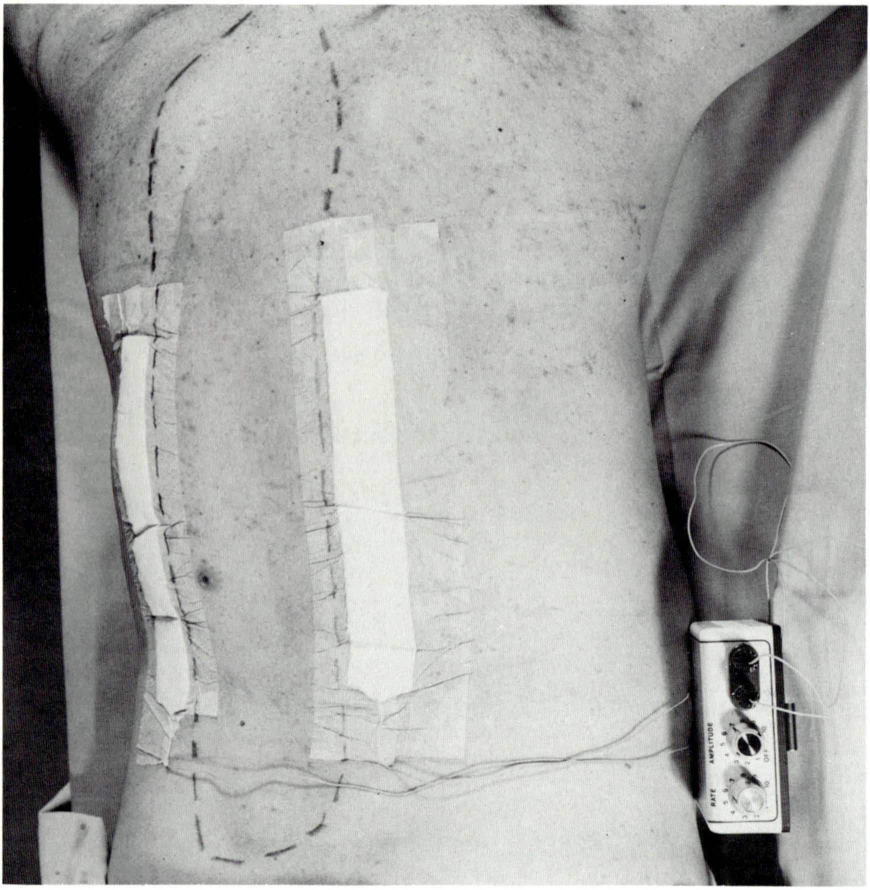

FIGURE 1. A patient, with mid-thoracic level paraplegia, is receiving TENS through modified, inexpensive entended electrodes. Pain relief was successful and he has used this combination for several years.

Chapter 12

TREATMENT OF THE MYOFASCIAL PAIN DYSFUNCTION SYNDROME WITH TRANSCUTANEOUS ELECTRICAL NEURO STIMULATION

MELVIN DENHOLTZ, D.D.S.

The dental profession has made great progress in the development of mechanical devices. Dentists can cast precision inlays, reshape a sagging face with plastic dentures, perform masterful and intricate works of total mouth rehabilitation, preserve teeth with sophisticated techniques of periodontal and root canal therapy. Crowns can be made which defy detection.

The elusive complaints of facial pain remain, despite technical advances. This pain is all the more baffling because it cannot be diagnosed using x-ray as can decay or an abcess. Because of the lack of visible pathology, dentists often dismiss this type of patient as a compulsive chronic complainer.

Most dental complaints can be handled with relative simplicity. We can cure a toothache. An infected nerve is easily pinpointed, but the vague, elusive pain of temporal mandibular joint and facial muscles does not have a clearly defined treatment.

We examined conventional methods of treating dental myofacial pain, as well as reviewing some of the less conventional modalities of treatment. These included behavior modification (1), psychotherapy (2), biofeedback (3), progressive relaxation (4), drug therapy (5), Myo-Monitor wave form stimulation (6), condylotomy (7), combined therapies including sympathy and reassurance (8), and T.E.N.S. (9).

The work done by Shealy and others with T.E.N.S. led us to examine Liss' work in this area (10). We utilized his device called the Pain Suppressor.TM. Basically, this battery operated pulse generator to which a pair of electrode tipped wires can be attached, providing mild, continuous electrical stimulation. For many, the pain signals traveling along the nerve pathways seem to be jammed before reaching the brain. This results in analgesia, often lasting long after stimulation ceases.

This device couples a 12 to 20 kilohertz waveform modulated by an 8 to 20 Hertz square wave at currents of 1 to 4 milliamperes to the site of pain, in our cases the masseter muscle or the temporal area, with electrodes. The current control is advanced until the patient is barely aware of a sensation of warmth, itching or flashing patches of light in the visual field. The current is then reduced just below the level of sensation. The initial period of treatment we used was 3 minutes. This might be extended in 3 minute intervals up to 30 minutes.

The theory of electrical nerve stimulation Liss adheres to in his studies is based on the following concepts:

1. Interference with the neural signs of pain at the sub cortical level in the centrum medianum of the thalmus.
2. Increase in blood flow by affecting the autonomic nervous system to bring increased oxygen and nutrients to the treated point of the body. The body then takes a finite time to return to its customary flow rate.

In one study of 20 patients suffering from myofacial pain dysfunction symptoms at Kimbrough Army Hospital, 16 patients reported "excellent," 2 reported "good," zero reported "fair" and 2 reported "poor" pain relief after stimulation. Of those aided by T.E.N.S., 40 percent felt relieved after a single application, while 90 percent were relieved after five applications.

Although most studies of the efficacy of T.E.N.S. were conducted on areas of muscular pain other than facial pain, we support its efficacy in this area as well.

At the Dental Research Department of the Newark Beth Israel Dental Health Care Center, a study is being made to evaluate T.E.N.S. using the Liss' device.

We have treated eleven patients with T.E.N.S., dividing them into two groups.

Group I was comprised of five patients who complained of sinus-type headaches (4 maxillary and 1 frontal sinus). These patients were undergoing routine dental care and had complained of these "headaches" just before routine dental work was about to be initiated. In each case, one electrode was placed on the pain site and the other at the web of the hand and Transcutaneous Electrical Neuro Stimulation was applied for periods of 3 to 6 minutes. After T.E.N.S. application was completed, the routine dental work was performed. The patients noted improvements in their "headaches" ranging from 50% to 90%, and all five seemed more relaxed and amenable to having dental work completed. This benefit alone can make T.E.N.S. an important adjunct to dental treatment.

Group II was made up of six patients exhibiting chronic histories of temporomandibular pain syndrome. These six were given a total of 114 applications of T.E.N.S., with each application period from 3 to 15 minutes duration. Each patient was given a unit to use at home daily, along with an evaluation sheet on which to chart their progress. Wide fluctuations of improvement were noted, ranging from zero to 90 percent, with a mean improvement of 37.5 percent.

Our study, although brief, seems to substantiate the theory that pain of short duration (such as headache) has a higher potential for improvement than chronic pain, which may be intertwined with emotional problems of long duration.

Since this was a cursory study, long term, accurate follow-up data of patients with chronic temporomandibular joint pain is still necessary. Preliminary data seems to justify Transcutaneous Stimulation as an adjunctive therapy, especially for those patients who have experienced failures with other modalities of treatment.

At the present time there is little evidence that T.E.N.S. is being widely used for dental purposes. Preliminary investigations indicate it will assume a more important role in the future of dentistry, such as in the treatment of localized osteitis, dental analgesia, dental anesthesia and alleviation of pain due to hot and cold sensitivity.

As stated, the syndrome known as Myofascial Pain Dysfunction may actually be a complex of many different etiological variants. Therefore, a treatment modality which works successfully for a given clinician or patient may not have any beneficial effects if applied under a new set of circumstances. This statement is made in light of research indicating that the specific physical form of therapy does not seem to be the essential factor in the determination of long-term success or failure in treatment of patients with MPD.

It therefore seems logical to use the more conservative of the previously noted analgesic modalities first, These, in conjunction with supportive communication techniques are preferable to over-treatment with radical or complex methods.

A review of the literature shows little published relative to the utilization of T.E.N.S. for the treatment of myofacial pain dysfunction. This exciting and important phenomenon seems to eradicate pain between the prescribed intervals of use. If, indeed, daily use of the device is required, then the degree of relief of pain must be weighed against its inherent inconvenience. But non-pharmacologic relief of pain is a tremendous advance.

The current research in this field shows much promise. Future research will, hopefully, shed more light on what is, at present, an incomplete understanding of the nature of Myofascial Pain Dysfunction, and the potential role T.E.N.S. may play in alleviating its related suffering.

BIBLIOGRAPHY

1. Gross, S.: Biofeedback technique in treating myo-fascial pain dysfunction syndrome. *J. N.J. Dent. Assoc.,46 (3)*:26-7, Spring 1975
2. Pomp, A.M.: Psychotherapy for the myofascial pain dysfunction syndrome: a study of factors coinciding with symptom remission. *JADA,89:*629-32 Sept. 1974
3. Carlsson, S., Gale, E., Ohman, A.: Treatment of temporomandibular joint syndrome with biofeedback training. *JADA,91*:602-5 Sept. 1975.
4. Gessel, A., Alderman, M.: Management of myofascial pain dysfunction syndrome of the temporomandibular joint by tension control training. *Psychosomatics,12*:302-9 Sept.-Oct. 1971.
5. Jagger, R.: Diazepam in the treatment of temporomandibular joint syndrome - A double blind study. *J. Dent.,2*:37-40 Oct. 1973.
6. Vesanen, E., Vesanen, R.: The Jankelson Myo-Monitor and its clinical use. *Proc. Finn. Dent.Soc.,69*:224-7 Dec. 1973
7. Tasanen, A., Von Konow, L.: Closed condylotomy in the treatment of idiopathic and traumatic pain-dysfunction syndrome of the temporomandibular joint. *Int.J.Oral Surg.,2*:102-6 1973.
8. Greene, C., Laskin, D.: Long-term evaluation of conservative treatment for myofascial pain-dysfunction syndrome. *JADA,89*:1365-8 Dec. 1974.
9. Shealy, C.N., Maurer, D.: Transcutaneous nerve stimulation for control of pain. *Surg Neurol.2(1)*:45-7 Jan. 1974.
10. Liss, S.: Copy of inventor's private research conducted at various institutions and clinics on the "pain suppressor" device.

Chapter 13

THE UTILIZATION OF T.E.N.S. IN A PRIMARY CARE HOSPITAL

ROBERT A. ERSEK, M.D.

To assess the adaptability of Transcutaneous Electrical Neuro Stimulation, we utilized it as a therapeutic modality as a primary means of affording pain relief for patients at Dover Air Force Base Hospital, Dover, Delaware. This is a primary facility, servicing 35,000 active duty personnel, dependents, and retired individuals.

The T.E.N.S. device was employed in the Emergency Department, General Surgery Clinic, and Surgical Ward during a six month period of time.

In the case of low back pain, referrals were made to the surgical service. Other orthopaedic cases also were referred there for treatment or transfer to orthopaedic centers. Additional cases were seen in the Surgical Out Patient Clinics, Emergency Department, or Surgical Ward, depending on where they were seen on initial referral. No attempt was made to isolate these patients or create a special environment for them. Other patients were treated at the same time in other rooms and wards.

All patients presenting with acute or chronic musculoskeletal pain were treated initially with T.E.N.S.

The study took place over a six-month period. Telephone follow-up was attempted on all patients. Three who were unavailable for follow-up were excluded from the study.

MATERIALS AND METHODS

The stimulator consists of a small 1x2.5x5.5 inch molded case which contains a rechargeable battery pack. The pulse frequency may be varied between 20-200 cycles per second. The pulse width ranges from between 0.1 msec to 1.0 msec Pulse amplitude may be varied from 9 to 120 volts. The maximum current output is 25 milliamps.

Three varieties of electrodes were used. A silicone rubber pad with a conductive surface adjacent to the patient was used most frequently. This pad was approximately 4 cm in diameter, with an outer non-conductive silicone rubber surface measuring approximately 7 cm in diameter. If irregular body contours were encountered, or more extensive areas of pain were present, a black conductive rubber strip electrode, measuring 1x9 inches was employed. For inpatients, where stimulation might be prolonged, a soft foam rubber disposable electrode with adhesive adjacent to the patient's surface was utilized. All of these electrodes are interchangeable, and have a universal snap coupling. When the electrodes were used on an out-patient basis, a disposable cotton swab was placed between the skin and the electrodes to insure maximum conduction with minimal resistance to the stimulating current.

Since this study, Davis (1) has described methods used to make electrodes with two-inch wide adhesive tape, self-adhesive Reston foam roll, No. 24 stranded insulated electrical hook-up wire, and aluminum-backed paper or aluminum foil. Several manufacturers now provide self-adherent electrodes.

To determine the area of electrode placement for obtaining optimum results, initially the patient described the area and quality of the pain to the physician or nurse in attendance. The electrodes were placed directly over the area where the pain was reported. Often, several different areas were stimulated during one treatment. Once the electrodes were placed in this area, the cotton alcohol swab was applied to the skin. The Gate Control Theory was briefly explained and the T.E.N.S. unit and each of the dials demonstrated. The patient then was prepared for the attachment of the electrodes. These were either taped or held by hand by the patient or technician prior to the application of any current. Understanding of the procedure to be undertaken reassured the patients, without engendering in them false hope for a "cure."

The T.E.N.S. dials were set with a pulse width of 4 and a rate setting of 4. No sensation is perceptible from the electrodes with the amplitude turned down to zero. Then the amplitude was gradually increased until the patient could definitely feel a light vibration. This might be achieved at a setting of 3 or 4, or, in the case of low back strain, the setting was at 5 or 6 before any perceptible vibration was noted.

When the patient reported the awareness of some slight vibration, the electrodes were moved, if necessary, to produce that vibration in the painful area. Once this was determined, the amplitude was increased gradually until the patient reported that it was quite definite. With very little training, a technician could soon adjust the amplitude to provide maximum vibratory sensation without eliciting nociceptor responses from overstimulation.

Frequently, the patient would be allowed to regulate the amplitude to achieve a level that was comfortable. The area again would be stimulated for five or ten minutes.

Again an estimate was sought of the percentage and degree of pain relief.

Then the intensity was decreased until no stimulation was perceptible. Another estimate of pain relief was sought.

The unit was then turned off, and the patient once again noted the amount of analgesia. If necessary, the electrodes were then placed in yet another area of pain and the same procedure repeated. The percentage rating of pain relief, while not ideal, is widely used (2).

Sternbach (3) discusses a method of measurement of pain whereby the patient tells when the pain matches his average pain and when it becomes unbearable. The latter is divided into former and multiplied by 100 to obtain the ratio expressed by the equation - tourniquet pain ratio equals:

$$\frac{\text{Average clinical pain (in seconds)}}{\text{Maximum tolerance time (in seconds)}} \times 100$$ - yielding a number from 0-100.

This can be compared to the pain estimate. In addition to the tourniquet test, activity measures and decreases in levels of analgesia reflect the patient's response and status.

Sternbach considers a two-week period of good results to

mean that stimulation is working effectively. Parenthetically, he also feels no patient should be excluded from treatment because of the Minnesota Multiphasic Inventory Score (M-MIS), a screening device used by some, as a chronic pain patient will generally have personality disorders (4).

CONTROLS

Each patient served as his own control during the evaluation and treatment. With a pulse width and rate setting of 4, an amplitude of zero, the amplitude was increased until the patient felt the vibration. If it was not felt in the pain area, the electrodes were moved until the patient very definitely felt vibration. He was at that point asked to evaluate the sensation and length of relief resulting from the stimulation. This gave the patient the opportunity of direct participation in the course of therapy.

RESULTS

During a six-month period in which 35 patients presented in the General Surgical Clinic or Surgical Ward with low back strain, all achieved from T.E.N.S. therapy what they described as at least a 50% reduction in their pain. The duration of symptoms ranged from a few hours to 20 years; the degree of injury or trauma varied from pain resulting from vacuum cleaning, to automobile accidents, followed by two laminectomies in previous years. In many cases of low back pain of acute onset, with no previous history, of this type of complaint, the relief of pain was prompt and permanent. In other cases where the low back pain was preceded by a long history of multiple operations and failure of analgesics and tranquilizers, the pain relief would vary between several hours and several days (5).

When we treated patients with this problem, T.E.N.S. therapy supplanted the previous mode of treatment of one to two weeks of strict bed rest, traction, analgesics and tranquilizers. (Figure I)

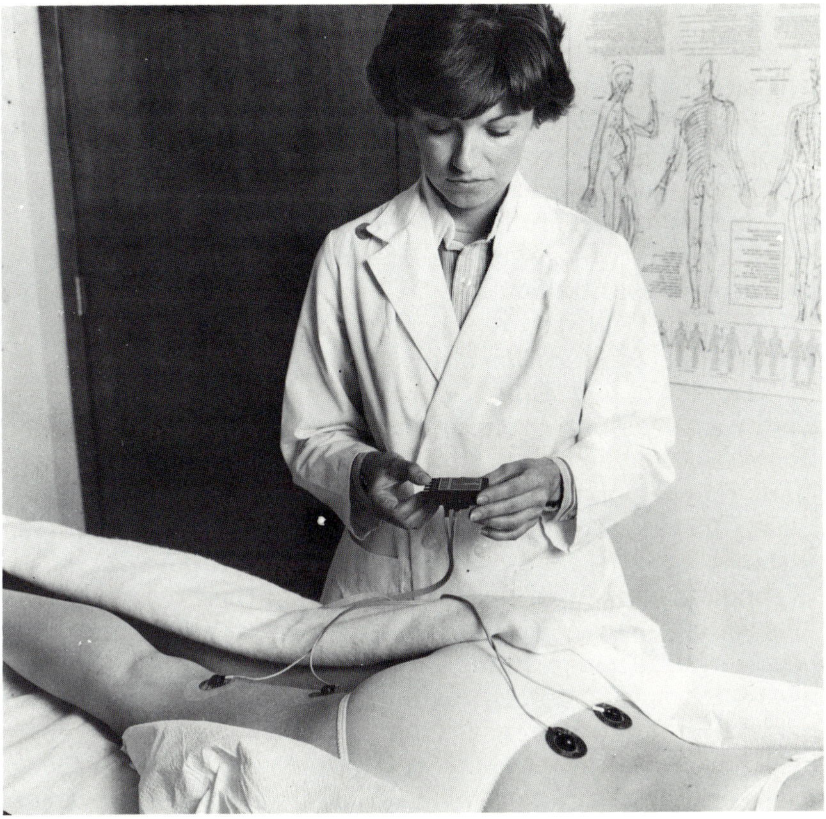

Shows placement or electrodes on a patient with Low Back Pain courtesy Med General

Many patients reported that when their pain recurred a few days later, it was less severe than it had been prior to T.E.N.S. treatment. Of those patients who had temporary relief, the minimum duration of reaction was three hours. Those who received relief lasting for hours or days were treated again in the same manner, and many continued to return to the clinic for periodic treatments with the T.E.N.S. unit every three days.

When the device was utilized more specifically in the Emergency Department with 34 patients with acute symptoms (lasting less than three days), six of these with acute pain symptoms were admitted to the hospital for their presenting symptoms of pain or other diagnoses, usually trauma. Only one of these received no pain relief, nine achieved what they reported as between 50-75 percent relief, six estimated between 76 and 89 percent relief, and eight between 90 and 99 percent, while ten attained 100 percent relief of their pain.

Seven patients presented with torticollis, or acute cervical strain. One patient with acute cervical pain secondary to an automobile accident experienced an increase in pain as a result of T.E.N.S. treatment. One achieved between 50 to 75 percent relief of pain, two over 90 percent relief, and three experienced 100 percent pain relief.

Figure II illustrates the percentage of relief afforded 51 patients included in this study.

The effect of T.E.N.S. in relieving pain and muscle spasm has often been very prompt and permanent. This is perhaps best shown in the cases of torticollis, where this form of treatment relieves pain, interrupting the pain-spasm-pain vicious cycle, allowing the patient full and voluntary control of his neck within a few seconds. Fifteen patients reporting on the telephone follow-up of this study said that their relief of pain or muscle spasm was permanent. One said the relief lasted 24 hours, and although some soreness returned, the patient still felt there was a 90 percent pain reduction. Another found some pain present on movement. This was a patient who had had low back strain following the lifting of boxes, who initially reported a 50 percent reduction in pain after T.E.N.S. treatment. Follow-up five months later revealed this patient still had some pain upon movement.

The patient presenting with shoulder and arm pain after lifting, initially reported 95 percent pain relief, and a follow-up report stated the relief lasted for ten days. One patient with recurring pain in the back following a fall, at first reported 80 percent reduction in pain, with relief lasting four days, and after a second treatment, relief was 100 percent and permanent. Another had relief for 48 hours, one for four days, another reported some soreness remaining.

CONCLUSIONS

Pain is an embarrassment to science. Although experienced by everyone to some degree, when it becomes debilitating in its acute or chronic states, there are vast socio-

PAIN RELIEF AFFORDED 51 PATIENTS USING TRANSCUTANEOUS NEURO-STIMULATION

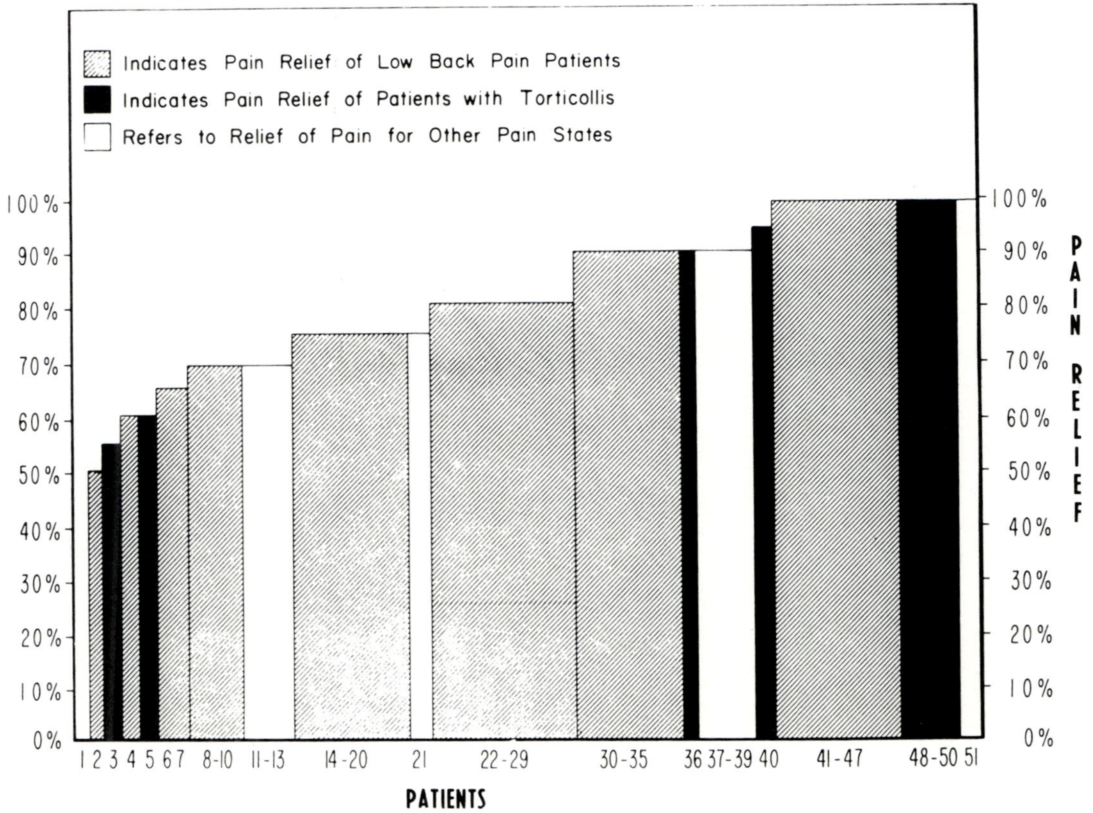

economic repercussions, affecting the physician, the patient, and those who inter-act with them.

Prior to the development and improvement of Transcutaneous Electrical Neuro Stimulating devices, pharmacologic therapy was the primary source of relief.

If suffering, even in a limited number of cases, can decrease, permit an individual to enjoy a more comfortable life, and free the physician to deal with other problems, Transcutaneous Electrical Neuro Stimulation will have proven its worth.

BIBLIOGRAPHY

1. Davis, R., Lentini, R.: Transcutaneous Nerve Stimulation for Treatment of Pain in Spinal Cord Injured Patients. *Bull. Prosth. Res.,298-301*, Fall, 1974
2. Cauthen, J.C., Renner, E. J.,: Transcutaneous and Peripheral Nerve Stimulation for Chronic Pain States. *Surg. Neurol.,4*:102-104, July, 1975.
3. Sternback, R.: Evaluation of Pain Relief. *Surg. Neurol.,4*:1990201, 1975.
4. Sternbach, R.: Psychological Aspects of Pain in the Selection of Patients. *Clin. Neuros. Proceed.* Congress of Neurol. Surg. Honolulu, 1973, Williams and Williams, 1974.
5. Ersek, R.A.: Low Back Pain, Prompt Relief with Transcutaneous Neuro-Stimulation. *Orthopaedic Rev.,5*:12:27-31, 1976.
6. Srivastave, K.P. and Saxena, A.K.: Electrical Stimulation in Delayed Union of Long Bones. *Orthopaedic Survey, 2* (3): 204, Nov.-Dec., 1978.
7. Endorphin Like to Pain Relief is Confirmed. *Medical World News, 88,* 93, February 19, 1979.
8. Stabile, Mark L. and Mallory, Thomas H., The Management of Postoperative Pain in Total Joint Replacement. *Orthopaedic Review, 7* (11): 121-123, November, 1978.
9. Pike, P.M.H.: Transcutaneous Electrical Stimulation: Its use in the management of postoperative pain. *Anaesthesia. 33:* 165-171, 1978.
10. Harvie, Keith W. Harvie: A Major Advance in the Control of Postoperative Knee Pain. *Orthopedics, 2* (1): 124-145, Jan./Feb., 1979.
11. Comper, Adrian: TENS, A New Dealer Market. *Surgical Business,* May, 1978.

Chapter 14

TRANSCUTANEOUS ELECTRICAL NEURO STIMULATION IN THE CONTROL OF CHRONIC PAIN

BOLESLAW RUTKOWSKI, M.D.

The problem of chronic pain control cannot be resolved by pharmacological means alone.

A real and ideal analgesic should fulfill the following requirements:

A. It should produce enough pain relief in various pathological conditions, and one dose of the drug should suffice for a long period of time.

B. It should be free from any undesirable side effects and be sufficiently effective even after continuous administration.

C. It should not be habit forming.

Of course, unfortunately, to date there is no such pharmacologic analgesia, and possibly it will never be produced.

Two other methods of dealing with pain are limited only to a few cases:

A. Blockades are restricted to some regions of the body and their effects are always of short duration.

B. Neurosurgery is connected with nervous destruction and loss of function.

The frequency of occurrence of chronic pain renders it not only a medical, but also a social and economic problem. It is an inseparable companion of many diseases, and when it is the chief, or only symptom, then it becomes the major disability. It is right and logical that it be treated. There are diseases, where from the start, there are no other symptoms except pain, such as trigeminal neuralgia or migraine.

Statistics offer us little valid information on how many patients are treated every year solely for pain. Records are simply not complete. Chronic recurrent headache is said to affect even 40% of the population. The incidence of migraine alone, according to various authors, ranges from 3 to 15% of the population.

Chronic low back pain affects individuals of all ages and it is estimated that in the United States, there are over six million persons who are being treated every year for that condition.

Rheumatic diseases are very common, and their importance need not be emphasized.

Although not all people with chronic pain seek medical advice and help, as in the cases with chronic recurrent headache, nevertheless, the crowd of those treated is increasing every year.

When pain is long lasting and intense, life becomes unbearable. All these patients are considered incurable cases, especially when all conventional methods of treatment have failed.

In our present time, we hear of new physical methods of pain control such as acupuncture, electroacupuncture, and electrical stimulation. Undoubtedly this last method thus far is the greatest achievement in current analgesia (Figure 1,2,3,).

According to various reports cited throughout the current literature, an appreciable percentage of patients with chronic pain will be treated by this method alone, without the need of any additional therapy.

Electrical stimulation is being performed in many ways, which may be broken into two main categories: transcutaneous electrical neuro stimulation and implanted electrode stimulation.

The first is gaining acceptance. It is simple, easy enough to be performed by any interested physician or his trained nurse, and, in many cases, by the patient himself at home. In the implanted method, the electrodes are implanted in the region of the spine or brain. This is, of course, a surgical method, applicable to very few cases.

Since 1972, electrical stimulation has been investigated, by our institution, using Transcutaneous Electrical Neuro Stimulation, or a modified method, with one transcutaneous electrode and two symmetrical needle electrodes. During this

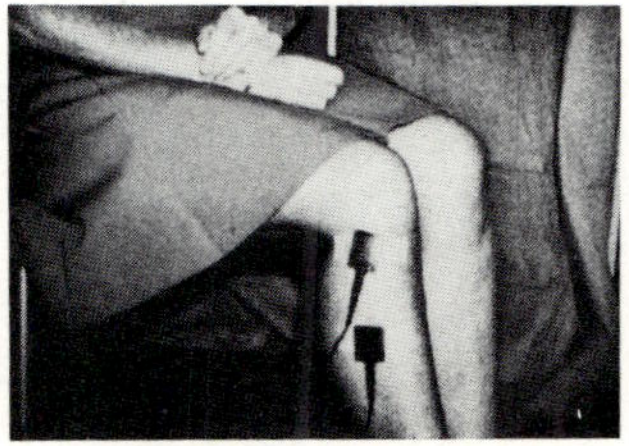

Neuralgic pain

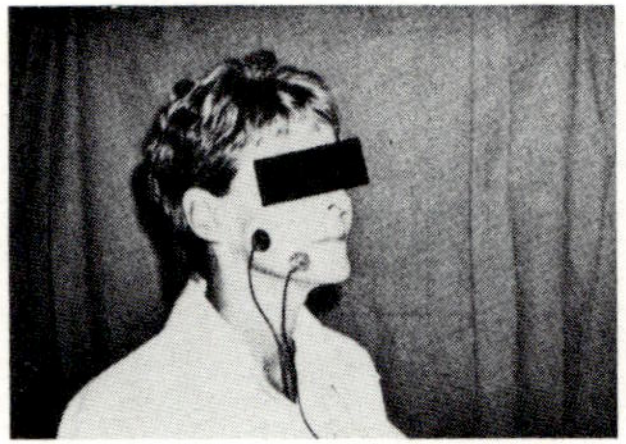

Atypical facial pain

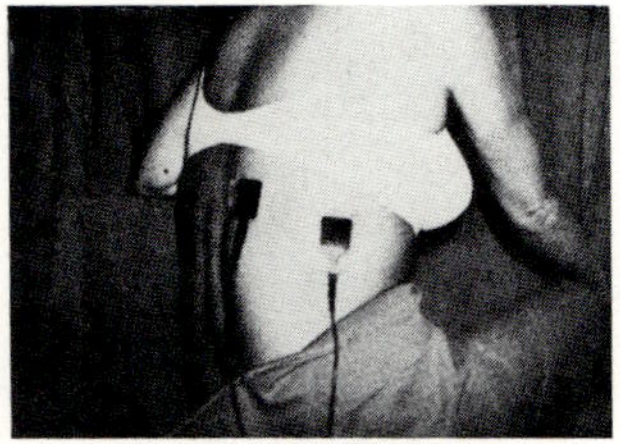

Intercostal neuralgia

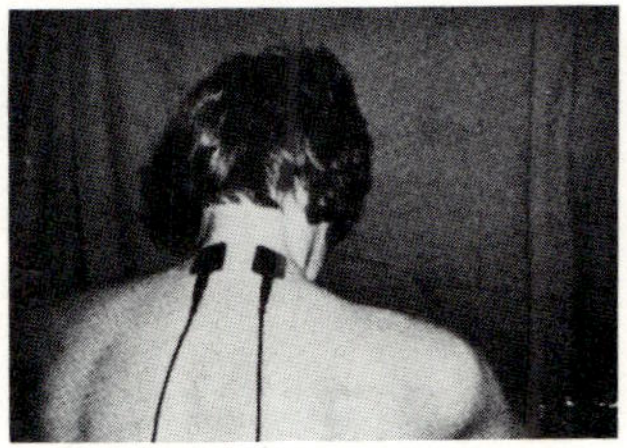

Neck pain

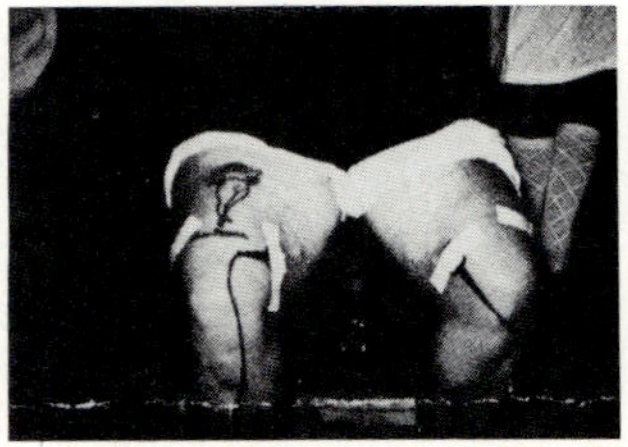

Reumatic pain

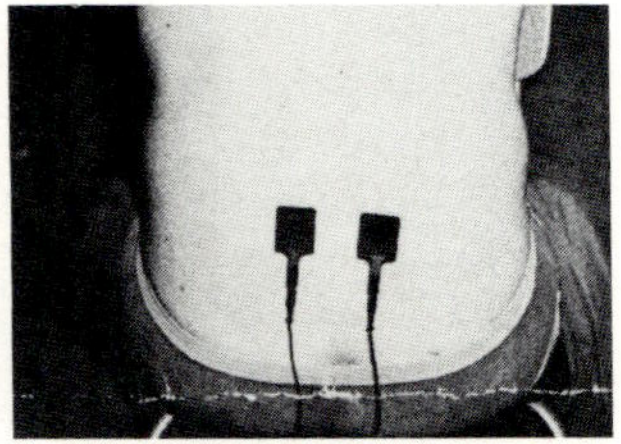

Chronic Lumbago

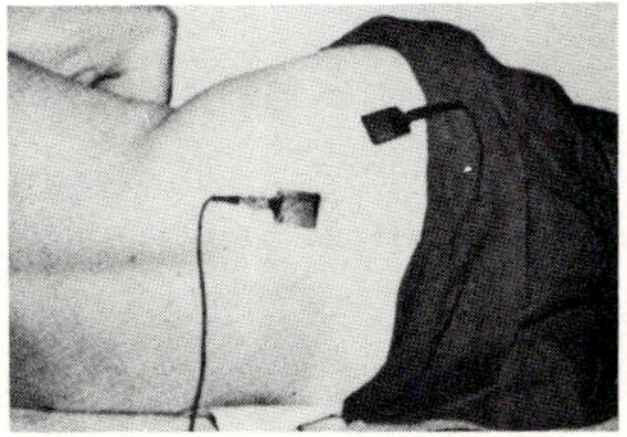

Chronic Lumbago with radicular pain

Credit Dan Sjö
Elektronik AB

Sundybyberg,
Sweden

period over 26,000 sessions on approximately 1500 patients have been performed.

The Method: The electrodes, contact (transcutaneous) or needles, were applied according to the localization of the pain. Thus, with the localization in the upper half of the body, two electrodes attached to a "Y" shaped wire were applied on both forearms and the circuit closed by another contact electrode placed in the interscapular region.

In pain of the lower half of the body, the two symmetrical electrodes attached to a "Y" shaped wire as above, were placed on the lateral aspect of both legs and the circuit closed by an electrode placed in either the interscapular or lumbar region.

The stimulator was linked to the alternative current from the network and was working on very low parameters.

In the case of needle electrodes, the parameters required were much lower because of the omission of skin resistance. A voltage of 0 to approximately 10 volts, and an intensity of 300-600 microamperes was sufficient. In Transcutaneous Electrical Neuro Stimulation, using only contact electrodes, higher parameters were necessary.

In the majority of cases, the shape of current was sine wave with a frequency of approximately 2 Hz, but also square and spike waves were used.

The application of the electrodes as described above could be changed according to the localization of the disease. Thus, in trigeminal neuralgia, instead of the interscapular region, the single third electrode was also placed on the jaw, either on the affected or opposite side.

In cases of chronic low back pain due to degenerative disc syndrome, apart from the two symmetrical electrodes in the legs, one or two additional electrodes were placed in the buttock of the affected side in the painful spots, which are easily found by pressing hard with the thumb, (the so called trigger points). If more than one such point is found, then a "Y" shaped wire is also used and attached by clips. This method of application is definitely better in cases of disc syndrome. If no painful or trigger points are found, the single electrode is placed as described above. (4)

In peripheral vascular disease, the electrodes should be placed as distally as possible. Thus, in Raynaud's disease, the electrodes were placed on the dorsum of both hands. In arteriosclerotic vascular disease of the lower extremities, and in Burger's disease as well, the electrodes were placed near the toes.

Sometimes in migraine, during an attack of pain, the single electrode was placed on the temporal region of the affected side.

All sessions of electrical stimulation were performed only in supine positions. Monitering of blood pressure and pulse is advisable, though not indispensable.

We have found 15 minutes to be the optimum time for stimulation. No less time achieves desired efficacy. Any appreciable prolongation of that period, though not detremental, did not significantly alter the effects.

The sessions were repeated according to the intensity of pain, every day or every other day for such a period, until evident improvement is obtained. Then the sessions are continued at a rate of once or twice weekly, or every fortnight indefinitely, as long as it is deemed necessary. This may continue for months, or even years. It has been our experience that some chronic cases were treated for two or more years, constituting more than one hundred sessions.

Results: This therapy is safe and free from any undesirable side effects in our series. The estimation of the results is based on the experience gained since 1972, with a follow-up of one to four years.

During the stimulation, the patient feels only a slight pulsatile sensation at the site of the electrodes. A few cases have complained of some slight dizziness of very short duration, just after the session.

Many of our patients stated that their sleep was improved and they usually feel much relieved.

In cases with hypertension, a significant fall of the systolic blood pressure was noted in the majority of observed patients.

According to the investigations performed, and our experience, the method is suitable for the treatment of following conditions:

A. *Chronic Recurrent Headache*. Under this heading, we included all types of chronic headaches of primary origin. The diagnosis of headache could be considered a challenge in the practice of medicine.

There are many classifications of this condition, but for the sake of experiments, the clinical classification was adopted as follows: classical migraine (mostly in women), cephalgia vasomotorica, cluster migraine, cervical syndrome (considered by some as secondary headache), and combined headache.

Classical migraine seems to be the most refactory for treatment. It is much easier to stop an attack of migraine, than to act prophylactically. An endocrinological factor is possibly involved. If the session is performed during the attack, one is likely to witness sudden, and even dramatic cessation of the pain. After many sessions, in 40% of cases, the attacks diminish in severity, duration, and frequency. Another 30% benefit to some degree from the stimulation, although their improvement is not so marked. In the remaining group, the condition remains unaltered.

Cephalgia vasomotorica is the most common type and often called just migraine. It affects men and women equally. The prodromal symptoms in this condition are less pronounced. The outlook is much better than in classical migraine, with the possibility of permanent remission. 50% of our patients responded favourably to TENS treatment.

Cluster headache is a rare condition, most common in men. It occurs usually at night, with excrutiating pain of the head, with no prodromes. This condition usually responds favourably to the therapy. The number of sessions is unlimited. Permanent remission could be expected. But there is the possibility of relapse after a year or two.

Cervical syndrome is a headache due, probably, to pathological changes of the cervical spine. The diagnosis usually is supported by an X-Ray evaluation. The outlook with stimulation is often favourable, after repeated sessions, and in some cases therapy must be continued indefinitely. Some 70% of our cases did benefit.

Combined headache presents a problem due to the fact that diagnosis is not certain, and even controversial. Psychological factors are involved. There still remains a category of patients where there is no specific diagnosis at all. At the start of the electrical stimulation, one can never be certain of the outcome of the treatment. It is, therefore, because of the minimal risk, valid to try this modality in all cases, when no other diagnosis was found.

There are, also, those patients who will complain of permanent headache, while its intensity is varying. They, too, may respond to this therapy.

It should be borne in mind that the treatment of headache is complex, and it must be directed to the whole person and not only his symptom. While this is applicable to all diseases, it is most true in headache.

One final remark regarding headache should be noted. The localization of the electrodes can be varied according to the condition. During an attack of migraine, as already mentioned, one electrode could be placed in the temporal region of the affected side. In cervical syndrome, when pain radiates to the neck and shoulder, the best sites for the electrodes are the tender, or trigger points of the neck or the suprascapular region, with two other electrodes on the forearms, as previously described.

B. *Primary Trigeminal Neuralgia*. This very common disease, with acute attacks of pain, usually unilateral (seldom bilateral), affects one or all three branches of the nerve. Patients, during their illness, are subjected to all types of therapy, i.e. drugs, blockades, alcoholization, and neurosurgery. All of these means are far from satisfactory and, in most cases, even after short remission, the attacks occur with the same severity. Some may complain of permanent pain, increasing with eating, speaking, washing the face, or tenderness on touch.

With electrical stimulation, the outlook for these cases is often favourable. In 40% of the cases, there is permanent remission of pain based on follow-up from a few months to 4 years, according to our studies. When relapses occur, they are treated in the same fashion. In the next 40%, there was also good response, i.e., the alleviation of pain was significant, there were fewer or less frequent attacks, but with some pain while eating continued to be a problem. The utilization of drugs was infrequent. Unfortunately, relapses were common. About 20% of these cases are refactory to the treatment, even after several sessions. Although some of them noted moderate alleviation of pain, these patients, in the unsuccessful group could not be deprived of their drugs.

From our experience we find the outlook better in younger individuals with shorter case histories, although this is not a hard and fast rule. Those patients who were already operated upon are often refractory. The same applies to those who complain of permanent pain.

We feel other neuralgias of the head could be treated in the same manner.

C. *Symptomatic Radiculitis*: Pain due to the diseases at all levels of the spine, such as spondylitis or degenerative disc syndrome can be categorized as being potentially aided by electrical stimulation.

Any conditions such as tuberculosis or tumors of the spine were not treated in this manner.

Radiculitis of the cervical region could be difficult to handle. Placement of the electrodes is better sought in the tender points of the suprascapular region. The percentage of those who will benefit is expected to be around 50%. The same applies to intercostal neuralgia.

The most difficult, for us, were the post-herpetic neuralgias.

In shoulder pain, any suspicion of osteo-arthritis must be excluded, since this is very difficult to treat.

The most promising results will be expected in chronic low back pain. When due to degenerative disc syndrome, the outlook could be as favourably high as 70%, with good to very good results. The sessions must be continued for weeks or months. Initially, with these patients, we begin first daily, then weekly, with some having twenty-five and more sessions, although the average was twelve to fifteen sessions. Though even dramatic results could be observed, only the final results were evaluated.

Low back pain due to spondylitis is more difficult to be treated, more sessions are necessary, and the treatment may sometimes be continued indefinitely. Nevertheless, some 50% of the cases in our study will not need any more drugs during the treatment.

Patients operated on for herniated disc responded well to the therapy.

D. *Pain Due to Peripheral Arterial Disease*: Conditions such as Raynaud's disease, Buerger's disease, and arteriosclerotic vascular disease of the lower extremities were included in the investigation. Intermittent claudication and other associated symptoms such as ulcerations and trophic changes of the skin were often improved. The treatment is continued with intervals indefinitely, and it is expected to last for years, so long as the patients benefit from it. In some cases, an evident improvement in the colour of the skin of toes, feet and legs can be observed. The effects may be expected after several sessions. Some patients, who could hardly walk without cramps in their legs for distances of thirty or forty yards, comment that during the treatment, the improvement is remarkable.

About 75% of all cases will benefit from T.E.N.S. therapy. Not only intermittent claudication or other pain can be improved, but also the ulcerations. The outlook is less favorable in diabetic cases.

E. *Neuralgias of Other Sites and Other Conditions*: Any neuralgia is a suitable case for the stimulation. Other conditions can also be treated, such as arterial hypertension, insomnia, neurasthenia, etc., subject to further experiments and investigation. The drop of the systolic blood pressure as observed in hypertonic patients, opens new possibilities in this field. This, as a rule, should be carried out in a ward rather than in outpatient departments.

F. *Intractable Cancer Pain*: This would constitute a separate chapter. Cancer cases with a life expectancy of months or years can be accepted into the program.

Those who were administered analgesics of the narcotic group previously for a long period are not suitable for this stimulation. This is self explanatory, and needs no additional comments. Of all cases with cancer pain, the best results were obtained with the following localizations: head and neck, and extremities, and sometimes in the spine. The abdominal localization was almost always refactory.

Stimulation may be continued indefinitely, as long as possible, along with any other forms of therapy of the disease.

G. *Rheumatic Diseases*: Not much experience was gained in rheumatic conditions. In rheumatoid arthritis, the treatment of pain while the swelling persists is useless. The same applies to cases with considerable anatomic damage of the joints such as degenerative osteo-arthritis of the hip and knee. Sometimes ankylosing spondylitis when associated with severe pain responds to treatment.

GENERAL CONSIDERATIONS AND CONCLUSIONS

At present, it is difficult to determine in what cases which kind of electrical stimulation will be the best. It is possible that this new modality for pain control is still in its initial stage. More experience must be gained and further research should be carried out. More research centres throughout the world must be involved.

The advantages of Transcutaneous Electrical Neuro Stimulation cannot be overemphasized. It is simple and safe. It can be performed by any physican or his trained nurse. It is applicable in a great variety of conditions, but the best results, according to our experience, can be obtained in neurological cases.

When needles are used as electrodes, electrical current of very low parameters can be applied, which is also very pleasant for the patient. Low frequencies were also adequate, since higher than 50 or 100 Hz did not improve the results.

The method gives a fair chance of pain relief for an indefinite period in an appreciable number of cases. Even cases considered as "incurables" can be satisfactorily treated.

To summarize, some points from our observations should be stressed:

1. There are some dramatic effects even after the first session, but the final results should be the purpose of the therapeutic process, not the immediate effect.

2. The alleviation of pain when observed, occurs after about 10-12 minutes of stimulation, and it may persist for several hours. This is also a sign that the outlook may be favorable. No less than three sessions have to be applied, if permanent results are to be expected.

3. No undesirable side effects were observed in our study, except for slight dizziness, usually in older or hypertensive patients, but this is transitory, and passes away before the patient leaves the surgery. In hypertensive patients, blood pressure should be monitored and recorded. The administration of antihypertensive drugs must be eventually stopped.

4. There is always a percentage of cases which will be refractory to electrical stimulation. Other methods of electrical

stimulation must be considered, or a combined therapy program instituted. Unfortunately, the problem of chronic pain control is far from being resolved.

5. There are chances of permanent relief in a number of cases with a follow up of months and years. After each series of sessions, the patient must be informed of his outlook in regard to his illness, and an adequate regime should be prescribed in all cases. In low back for instance, the patient would be instructed how to take care of his spine and some light physical training may be advisable.

6. In cases where there is not complete remission of the symptoms, the treatment can be continued indefinitely, usually with intervals between the series of sessions. The physician will decide as to the length of the interval. So long as the patient benefits from the therapy, there is no limit of time and number of sessions to be applied. If relapses of pain should occur, as seen in trigeminal neuralgia or low back pain, the treatment will be performed as before, with the same expectation.

7. Possibly, more valuable experience will be gained, if electrical stimulation utilized and reported on by a larger number of medical practitioners, finds its place in the literature, so that the pros and cons of this relatively new method of pain diminution or alleviation may be more clearly understood.

References

1. Melzack, R. Wall, P.D. (1965) Pain Mechar isms: A New theory. Sceince, 150, 971
2. Oliveras, J.L., Besson, J.M., Guilbaud, G., Liebeskind, J.C. (1974). Behavioral and electrophysiological evidence of pain inhibition from Mid-Brain Stimulation. Exp. Brain Res., 20, 32.
3. Wall, P.D., Gutnick, M. (1974) Properties of afferent nerve impulses originating from a Neuroma. Nature (Lond.) 248, 740
4. Ruthkowski B., Niedzialkowska, T., Otto, J. Electrical Stimulation in Chronic Low Back Pain. Br. J. Anaesth. (1977) 49, 629

Chapter 15

TRANSCUTANEOUS ELECTRICAL NEURO STIMULATION IN THE ASSESSMENT OF PATIENTS FOR ELECTRICAL STIMULATOR IMPLANT

JOHN MILES, M.B., B.Ch., F.R.C.S.

Counter irritation as a means of relieving pain is of untold antiquity; in its most simple form of rubbing the injured spot, it is presumably an innate animal behavioral act. Primitive cultures have sometimes developed exotic and even flamboyant methods of counter irritation (Fig. 1). Electricity in the form of the defensive electric shock produced by certain fish such as the torpedo fish, has been used in the treatment of painful disorders and presumably with some success.

In the nineteenth century, generated electricity was rapidly incorporated into routine medical practice with analgesic and also primary therapeutic intention (Fig. 2). Interestingly, one of the first two patients subjected, by Abbe (1), to sensory root section for his pain, was reported to have previously failed to respond to electrical stimulation. Gross malpractice ensured the early exclusion of electro-therapy from general medical practice except in certain aspects of physical medicine.

In 1965, Melzack and Wall (2), on the basis of animal experiments developed the Gate Contol Theory to explain the pain relief apparently occurring in these animals during electrical stimulation. Wall and Sweet (3) applied the same principle in experiments on themselves and this rapidly led on to the

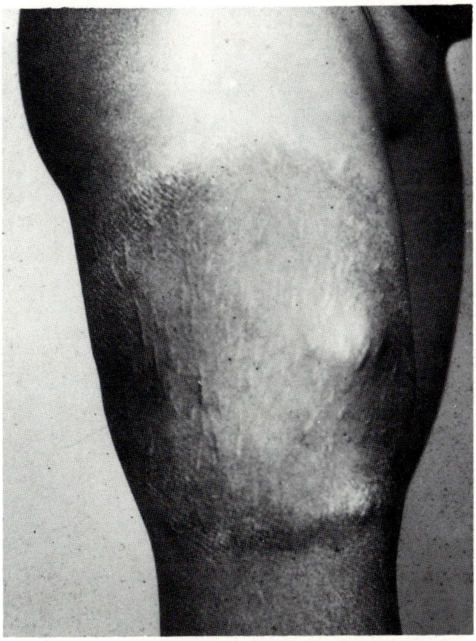

Figure 1. Scarification of the skin, a primitive form of counter-irritation.

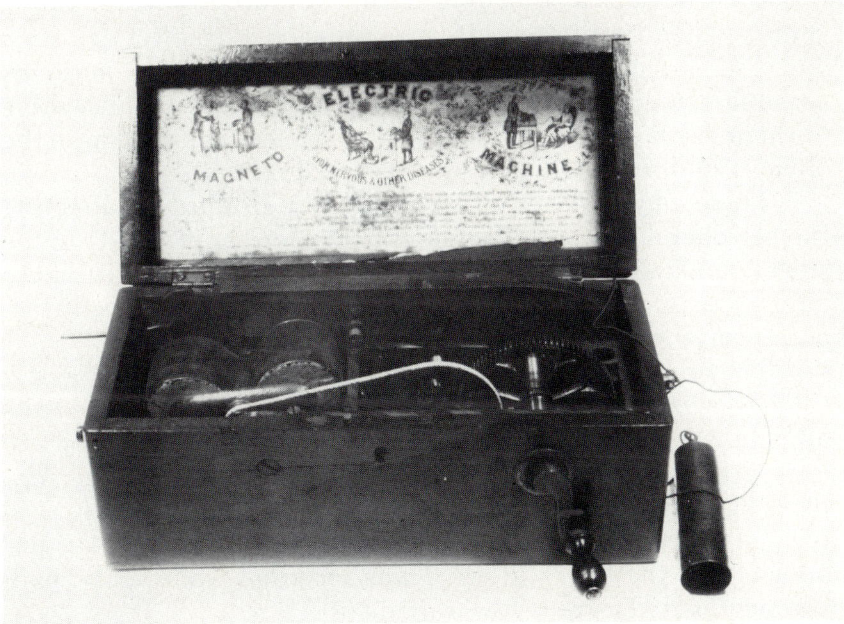

Figure 2. Early, hand driven, electrical stimulator "for Nervous and other Diseases." (Courtesy Dr. Gwyn o Denbych.)

widespread, respectable and credible application of electricity for pain relief.

Shealy described the implantation of an electrode onto the posterior columns of a patient suffering pain due to cancer and how continuing stimulation could be achieved by the use of an implanted receiver activated through the skin by a transmitter controlled by the patient (4). Shealy, Sweet and Nashold entered the new field of implanted electrodes with enthusiasm and early reports of initial success in cases known to be resistant to conventional methods, encouraged others (5,6,7). Initially, implantation was on the basis of diagnosis but quite rapidly it became obvious that this form of selection was not good enough. Electrical stimulation was clearly not able to suppress all pain.

Two of the first three patients on whom I implanted dorsal column stimulators obtained no relief from their pain, though each had a respectable and well recognized chronic pain syndrome, examples of which had been treated effectively by this method by others. Assessment of suitability for this form of treatment was clearly going to be the main problem.

On the basis that electrical stimulation was but a sophisticated twentieth century expression of counter irritation our assessment protocol was designed to include as many as possible examples of physical interference, either provocative or therapeutic to the pain. This was of course in addition to the obvious and vital criteria indicated in Figure 3.

These physical activities have been grouped as affecting the peripheral nerve, the segment of the cord appropriate to the site of pain and the posterior columns cephalad to the site of the pain. The groupings cannot be considered scientifically accurate save perhaps the first.

The effect on the pain by each test has been graded as 2 if there was excellent relief, so that during the period of the tests all pain was suppressed. Partial relief, grade 1, was said to have been attained if the pain at its worst broke through the suppressing influence of the test or if the pain, though totally suppressed in some areas continued in others. If the pain was unaffected by the test a grade 0 was recorded while if the pain was aggravated a grade X was made (8).

Figure 3

ASSESSMENT PROTOCOL

Clinical	
Pharmacological	
Psychiatric	
Physiological	
	- Sensory thresholds
	- Cerebral evoked potential
Provocative	
	- Peripheral Nerve
Abrasion	
Transcutaneous Electrical Stimulation	
Precutaneous Electrical Stimulation	
	- Segment of Cord
Acupuncture	
Interspinous Ligament Injection	
	- Posterior Columns
Extradural Percutaneous Electrical Stimulation	
Subarachnoid Percutaneous Electrical Stimulation	

TECHNIQUE

In the evaluation of patients' suitability for stimulator implant, except for abrasion, by rubbing of available peripheral nerves, transcutaneous electrical neuro stimulation must be, at least in principle, the simplest test. While nerve abrasion requires no equipment, it is really limited to syndromes in which pain is localised to specific nerve distributions and in which the peripheral nerves are easily palpable.

Transcutaneous Electrical Neuro Stimulation has several definite advantages when compared with other tests. It is non-invasive and suffers few complications. Save for an infrequent occurrence of allergic reactions to electrode contact fluid, the only risk is that of an electrical skin burn occurring when excessive electrical stimulation has been applied to a denervated or poorly inervated area of skin. Such a risk is definitely present in patients suffering from post herpetic neuralgia.

As a test procedure, Transcutaneous Electrical Neuro Stimulation is extremely flexible and as long as the observer has sufficient time to devote to the investigation, it allows of infinite exploration into the effect of electrical stimulation. This is important as it is by no means established which sites are best stimulated in order to achieve maximal pain relief.

It does appear clear that stimulation in totally anaesthetic areas has no worthwhile effect and as mentioned carries some risk. Stimulation can be made directly over the site of pain or over the expected sites of the nerve trunk supplying the area of pain. Although it is said (Thoden, 1976 (9)) to make no therapeutic difference, I personally find stimulation of the supplying nerve to be associated with a more definite and clear cut response than stimulating over the area or areas of pain.

Areas remote from the pain and the nerve supplying the painful areas have also been found to be effective in relieving pain (Laitinan, 1976 (10)). As with perhaps no other test, Transcutaneous Electrical Neuro Stimulation is suitable for exploring this possibility.

Transcutaneous Electrical Neuro Stimulation can be repeated and the result is even more convincing if it occurs after a definite interval of time. Equivocal responses can be reassessed and conclusions reached.

Transcutaneous Electrical Neuro Stimulation can be used over a prolonged period and this engenders several other advantages. Paraesthesiae produced by Transcutaneous Electrical Neuro Stimulation, while not always absolutely reproducing the sensation of an implanted electrical stimulator, simulates the sensation to a sufficient degree as to allow the patient to decide on its acceptability. This aspect is, I believe, not too difficult a consideration, as in my experience the patients getting the best pain relief often describe the paraesthesiae in clear cut terms of pleasurable sensation, quite different a description from that used by the patients who are not getting much pain relief. The description of 'pleasant' as opposed to pricking paraesthesiae has made Dr. Albe-Fessard believe that in these instances the effect of stimulation relates to a level higher than the peripheral nerve and cord. She believes that the sensation obtained by stimulating the peripheral nerve or the cord is of a rather unpleasant pricking quality. This is obviously not the place to explore this interesting hypothesis.

More frequently, prolonged testing is a reflection and obligation of uncertainty in the objective assessment. In cases such as phantom arm pain, it is easy to be certain of accurate electrode placement over the nerve trunks in the stump and therefore to be sure of major or maximal stimulation. In phantom leg pain, the sciatic nerve is not as easily felt and with the great bulk of tissue in the stump, maximal stimulation by specific electrode placement is by no means as sure. In such circumstances, I tend to place the electrodes in line with the expected anatomical position of the nerve with the upper being placed midway between the femoral greater trocanter laterally and the ischial tuberosity medially, in the lower third of the buttock. The lower electrode is then placed distally and at least initially is placed either laterally or medially depending on whether the complaint of pain is in the distribution of the lateral or medial popliteal nerves.

Less discrete areas of pain such as on the trunk, especially over the back, allow of much more uncertainty regarding optimal placement and effect and subsequently benefit from and require prolonged testing.

It is particularly in these circumstances that a range or variety of electrodes proves useful. Whereas simple button electrodes are satisfactory for stimulating a palpable nerve, larger electrodes, shaped electrodes and strip electrodes as illustrated in Figure 4, are often more effective in obtaining a response in anatomically awkward or extensive areas of pain.

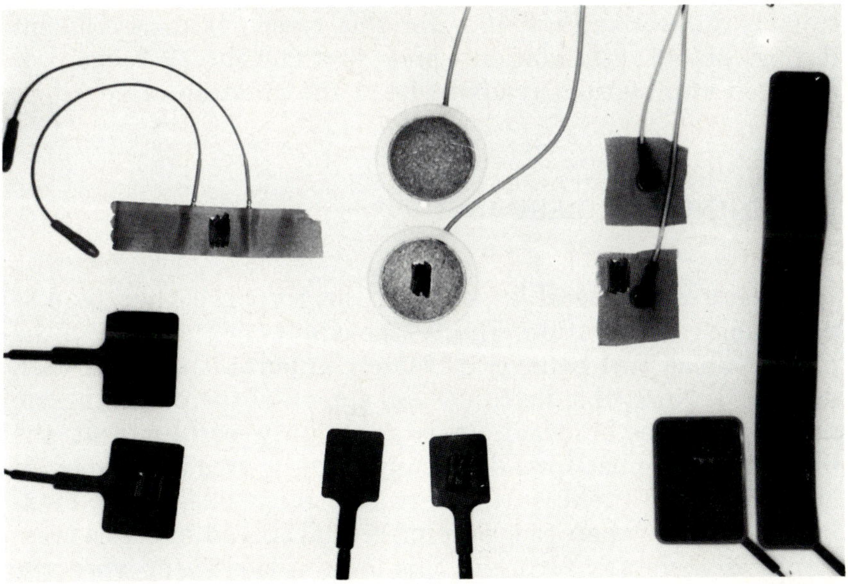

Figure 4. Some of the Electrodes available for Transcutaneous Electrical Stimulation.

Another very definite value of Transcutaneous Electrical Neuro Stimulation is the protracted period of testing that can be achieved, so that the test can be continued out of the protected environment of the hospital and in the more complex milieu of normal life. Invariably, patients with chronic pain syndromes, even when these have been present for more than thirty years, state that they get noticably less pain during hospitalization. Whether this is the effect of removing the patient from the stressful problems of everyday life or whether it is a positive response to the attention that he gets while in hospital, it leaves a very definite possibility that thorough and complete testing of the efficacy of electrical stimulation can only occur out of hospital.

It is, however, not simply a matter of sending the patient away with instructions of 'explore all areas and electrode combinations.' This management at least with our patients has proved almost invariably futile, even when the patient's intellect might have been expected easily sufficient to the task. No, unfortunately, assessment by T.E.N.S. usually demands a great deal of skilled observer time and when the stimulation is a prologue to surgical implantation this usually means by the surgeon himself, or one of his close and responsible associates.

Interpretation of the effect, of necessity, tends to be extremely subjective, and it is for this reason that assessment during actual stimulation, and particularly prolonged or repeated stimulation, tends to be of the greatest value.

ASSESSING THE RESPONSE

There are several aspects of the response that require particular consideration. Firstly, the quality or character of the paraesthesiae is, I believe, extremely important and has been described. Next, the distributional spread of the paraesthesiae needs to be established. It is now fairly certain that the paraesthesiae must spread strongly into the area of the pain in order to obtain therapeutic effect and this is likely to be maximal only when there is even preferential spread into this area. Rarely is there any future to this form of treatment when the painful area receives no paraesthesiae. Not infrequently the paraesthesiae spread incompletely into the painful area and some pain persists. It is very easy for the patient during the first experience of the test to misinterpret the detail of the spread and time must be allowed for greater accuracy. A classical example of this is for a patient with phantom limb pain to note the rapid spread of the paraesthesiae, resulting from Transcutaneous Electrical Neuro Stimulation, into the phantom limb but only later to realize that it in fact never passed into the digit of maximal pain. We had to learn, through failure, that this meant that implantation was contra-indicated.

The assessment can be improved by cross-questioning the patient. Did the paraesthesiae mix in with their pain or do the two sensations remain separate? Undoubtedly intimate mixing is associated with more effective pain relief. If it does not, does the paraesthesiae seem in any way to be interfering with the pain? Lastly, does the patient recognize any distracting affect as a result of the paraesthesiae? These extremely leading questions seem necessary in the difficult matter of interpreting the therapeutic effect of electrical stimulation.

RESULTS (Fig. 5)

No single test is so reliable as to predict with absolute surety the success of implanting a stimulator. The effect of acupuncture delivered either on a dermatomal or a meridian basis, has, throughout our study, been slight and of no value in assessment. Otherwise, it has been a matter of correlating the responses to several tests in order to decide on implantation.

When the response has been repeatedly excellent the decision is obvious. Similiarly, if the simpler tests such as nerve abrasion and Transcutaneous Electrical Neuro Stimulation have been unequivocally encouraging then implantation has been undertaken without proceeding to more complex tests. One of our patients with phantom arm pain illustrates this point. He obtained excellent relief of his pain by abrasion of the nerves in his stump and equally good relief by Transcutaneous Electrical Neuro Stimulation to the stump. As all features in his history and examination including the possession of an extremely reliable and stable personality were in favour, a

Figure 5. *RESULTS:*
37 patients with chronic pain syndromes.
33 patients with satisfactory transcutaneous electrical stimulation testing.

Test grading in 33 patients:

(2) - 9
(1) - 11
(0) - 12
(X) - 1

Results of implantation related to test grading:

Test grading (2)

9 patients
6 implanted
3 maintained on transcutaneous electrical stimulation

Results on Implantation:

(2) - 4
(1) - 2
(0) - 0
(X) - 0

Test grading (1) -

11 patients
8 implanted
3 not, -1 because of conflicting results.
-1 because of poor radiation of paraesthesiae
-1 did not complete his assessment

Results on Implantation:

(2) - 3
(1) - 5
(0) - 0

Test grading (0) -

12 patients
6 implanted
1 removed because of infection

Results on Implantation

(2) - 0
(1) - 3
(0) - 2
(X) - 0

Test grading (X) -

1 patient
implanted when assessment criteria were unclear

Results on Implantation

(2) - 0
(1) - 0
(0) - 1
(X) - 0

Test gradings and results are classified as

(2) - Excellent
(1) - Some Relief
(0) - No Relief
(X) - Aggravation

stimulator was implanted on the peripheral nerves in the stump with the anticipated and excellent result and this has continued, now, for four years. If during the tests the pain is aggravated (X) or there is no effect (0), then again the decision is obvious and no implantation to the peripheral nerve or posterior column is undertaken.

There is still the problem of the large group of patients who obtain some relief of pain but who have a 'mixed bag' result with the grades of response to the various test ranging from 0 to 2. It is then that other factors attain crucial importance in making the decision for implantation. Undoubtedly the personality of the patient is the single most important consideration.

In this respect, the development of a form of psychological dependence on the pain syndrome, over the period of its duration, must be carefully considered. The presence of continuing litigation or compensation relating to the cause of the pain is always a serious threat to the success of therapy and in these circumstances weighs heavily against implantation. A history of drug dependence, likewise, is an added threat to the success of any treatment. Whereas in the situation of unequivocally good responses to tests and apparently satisfactory withdrawal from such drugs, there is still the possibility of implantation, in the equivocal response group this would perhaps dissuade the surgeon.

The less easily defined influence that partially relieving the pain might have on the patients lifestyle, in particular his work is also important. If just twenty percent pain relief allowed him to re-establish himself in his family or in his work or in his life outside work it would be worthwhile implanting a stimulator to achieve this. If, however, for whatever reason, partial relief of pain seems unlikely to prove sufficient a foundation on which to build a rehabilitation, then implantation is not to be advised. This decision is always difficult.

CONCLUSION

The assessment of a patient's suitability for stimulator implant as a means of relieving chronic pain is not as simple or certain as was hoped. In many circumstances, it remains an opinion based on multiple and equivocal indicators. In cases of great responsiveness, Transcutaneous Electrical Neuro Stimulation is usually positive and unequivocal and obviates more invasive tests such as percutaneous indwelling electrodes. In too many situations, however, Transcutaneous Electrical Neuro Stimulation appears, for technical reasons, ineffective and yet significant relief can be obtained by electrical stimulator implant.

Transcutaneous Electrical Neuro Stimulation is harmless and though time-consuming and often demanding of the medical advisor, can be used repeatedly and over periods prolonged enough to give considerable confidence to the decision making.

REFERENCES

1. Abbe, R., (1889): A Contribution to the Surgery of the Spine. *Med. Rec. (N.Y.),35:*149-152.
2. Melzack, R., Wall, P.D. (1965): Pain Mechanism : A New Theory. *Science,150*:971-9.
3. Wall, P.D., Sweet, W.H. (1967): Temporary Abolition of Pain in Man. *Science,155*:108-9.
4. Shealy, C.N., Mortimer, J.T., Reswick, J.B. (1967): Electrical Inhibition of Pain by Stimulation of the Dorsal Columns. *Anaesth. Analg. curr. Res.,46*:489-491.
5. Shealy, C.N., Mortimer, J.T., Hagfors, NR. (1970): Dorsal Column Electroanalgesia. *J. Neurosurg.,32*:560-4.
6. Nashold, B.S., Friedman, H. (1972): Dorsal Column Stimulation for Control of Pain. *J. Neurosurg.,36*:590-7.
7. Sweet, W.H., Wepsic, J.G., (1973): *Electrical Stimulation for Suppression of Pain in Man.* In Fields, W.S. (ed): *Neural Organisation and its Relevance to Prosthetics.* New York. Intercontinental Medical Book Corp. pp. 219-240.
8. Miles, J., Hayward, K., Mumford, J., Lipton, S., Bowsher, D., Molony, V. (1974): Pain Relief by Implanted Electrical Stimulators. *Lancet, i,* 777-9.
9. Thoden, U. (1976): Results of Transcutaneous Electrical Stimulation. Presented to the 2nd Symposium on Electrical Stimulation. Davos, Switzerland 10th-11th December, 1976.
10. Laitinan, L. (1976): Should we stimulate the painful area or the healthy side of the body. Presented to the 2nd Symposium on Electrical Stimulation. Davos, Switzerland, 10th-11th December, 1976.

Chapter 16

THE USE OF ELECTRICAL IMPULSES APPLIED TO THE SKIN FOR RELIEF OF PAIN

WALTER INDECK, M.D.

The patient who is beset with a condition associated with chronic pain creates ever increasing concentric circles of "involvement."

The core and central circle is a patient who becomes frustrated by repetitive visits to his physician, multiple discipline consultations, frequent hospitalizations, and occasional repeated surgical procedures.

The circle enlarges to involve the immediate family and friends, obligating them to balance the problem of being sympathetic to the patient's demands and yet not "contributing to a vicious cycle" by accommodating the every wish of the "ailing one."

The circle finally expands to include the family physicians who become frustrated with the inability, at times, to cope with the apparent persistence of excruciating pain, continued disability and the added problems of complex emotional factors.

The ever increasing numbers of pain clinics in both inpatient and outpatient configuration attest to the professional awareness of the importance of these conditions. Constructive programs have been created to cope with the multifaceted problems.

The all-encompassing circle is the economic problem created by the sequel to the patient's inability to be gainfully employed, industry's concern in modifying jobs to accept such individuals, and the all-important drain through insurance programs to maintain this individual through physician, surgeon and hospital care costs.

Whatever alternatives can be made that can substitute for inpatient supervision and non-invasive procedures offer great advantages for both patient and physician supervision.

Such a non-invasive, well-tolerated and effective technique is the use of battery generated electrical impulses for the relief of pain.

Whenever pain pathways can be suspended, even temporarily, there frequently occurs an unexplained long-lasting effect of this relief. Injection of trigger zones with a local anesthetic is an excellent example of the success of this correlation.

Possibly, because pain is so poorly understood, there are many theories offered to explain the initiation of this sensation and its subsequent perception within the brain.

A popular hypothesis, in the past, has been the specificity theory. Here, free nerve endings in the skin have been identified as possibly transmitting impulses through specific tracts centrally. How extremes of temperature are interpreted as painful stimuli becomes difficult to explain on a specificity theory basis, and conversely, areas in which only free pain nerve endings are identified, may be associated with the ability to detect temperature changes!

It has been suggested that once a stimulus is applied to the skin a particular "pattern" is created in a sequence that is interpreted through past experience by the brain. These "patterns" would then explain the extremes of temperature creating painful responses but would not explain the modifying emotional factors that can inhibit or exaggerate specific pain "patterns."

In the past decade, the "gate control" hypothesis has helped to explain some of the possible effects of the electrical impulses in diminishing the perception of pain.

The hypothesis has had many modifications in respect to refinement of the original thesis and many challenges in respect to clinical practice. It does, however, serve as a possible answer to the efficacy of battery generated impulses.

There may be several ways in which pain can be modified as explained by this theory. Large and small fibers have varying effects on the transmission and perception of pain. If a large fiber is stimulated, a "gate is closed" and there apparently results a blockade of the pain impulse. Small fiber stimulation tends to "open the gate" and allow perception of pain.

The gate control also is attractive in that it could possibly explain descending impulses from the brain acting in a similar fashion as large fiber stimulation and thereby inhibiting the perception of pain. This emotional "modifier" can explain the apparent insensitivity of some patients using voluntary control to diminish the intensity of painful stimuli, Other "gate" control sites may be present throughout the spinal cord and brain stem areas to add to these modifying impulses. Some authors have postulated the central gray area of the brain stem to be capable of inhibiting pain. It has been suggested that impulses peripherally initiated would produce brain stem inhibitory fiber activation which would then block pain signals from other areas.

The intense output of impulses generated by the unit might act by disrupting reflex cycle chains either by inhibiting the perpetuation at spinal level or indirectly by activation of the brain stem inhibitory mechanisms.

It is this cycle, once broken, that might explain the clinical prolonged effects of a single injection of an anesthetic into the trigger zone about a nerve site or the use of acupuncture needles in specific areas.

STIMULATORS

The use of electrical stimulators in an effort to block pain impulses was encouraged by the early clinical results obtained when units were applied to the skin of patients experiencing chronic pain. Neither the nerve ending nor the pathway transmission tracts apparently could correctly identify one impulse that was initiated by a painful stimulus from another impulse that was generated by a battery. Early reports attested to the efficacy in diminishing the perception of pain and various stimulators were designed to initiate this impulse.

The instruments basically provide control of voltage, frequency and type of pulse initiated. The currents generated by the units were extremely low and almost uniformly well tolerated by the patients. Whenever the electrodes were applied near a painful area, pain relief was usually obtained. In some instances, where large areas of trigger zones existed, multiple dermatome segments could be "crossed" by extending electrode application adjacent to the spine to overlay successive segments.

At times, relief is complete, dramatic and will continue even after the battery generated impulses are discontinued. This "after effect" is extremely variable but also important to the patient in that constant application of the current is not necessary.

Several investigators have used the external stimulation as a diagnostic tool inasmuch as it can serve as a screen for patients who might ultimately benefit from a similar electrical device implanted adjacent to the dura in an effort to more completely block the ascending pathways in the dorsal columns.

The use of the external device must be thoroughly explained to the patient and it is this aspect of consideration that is sometimes minimized in the entire program.

Frequently, changes in the area of application are necessary in an effort to obtain the most effective blockade pattern.

TECHNIQUE OF APPLICATION

An important factor contributing to the success of the application of electrical impulses is the thorough training given to the patient by trained personnel. This initial training and time is necessary in order to allay the patient's fears as well as encourage confidence in the patient so that he can change the position of the electrodes to enhance the effectiveness.

The initial introduction of the patient to the device should be the application of an electrode to a non-painful area such as the back of the forearm. Once applied, the patient is familiar with the sensation of electrical stimulation which usually consists of the sensation of vibration at the lower voltages.

As the voltage is increased a painful sensation and "biting" may occur at which point the output is decreased until a non-painful stimulus is easily accepted.

Impulse frequency and duration can also be varied until the "ideal" is found to the patient's tolerance. Areas with less subcutaneous tissue overlying bony prominences accept lower thresholds than less tactfully supplied areas such as the low back and buttock.

The electrode placement is usually initiated overlying the painful area (Figure 1, 2 and 3) and if this is ineffective in relieving symptoms more proximal placement can be tried in an effort to block ascending painful impulses. Remote areas of application appear to be more successful during the introduction of acupuncture techniques than when applied with the transcutaneous electrode.

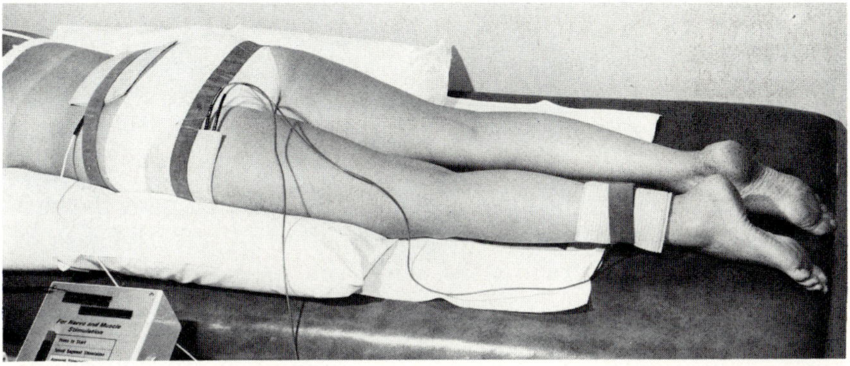

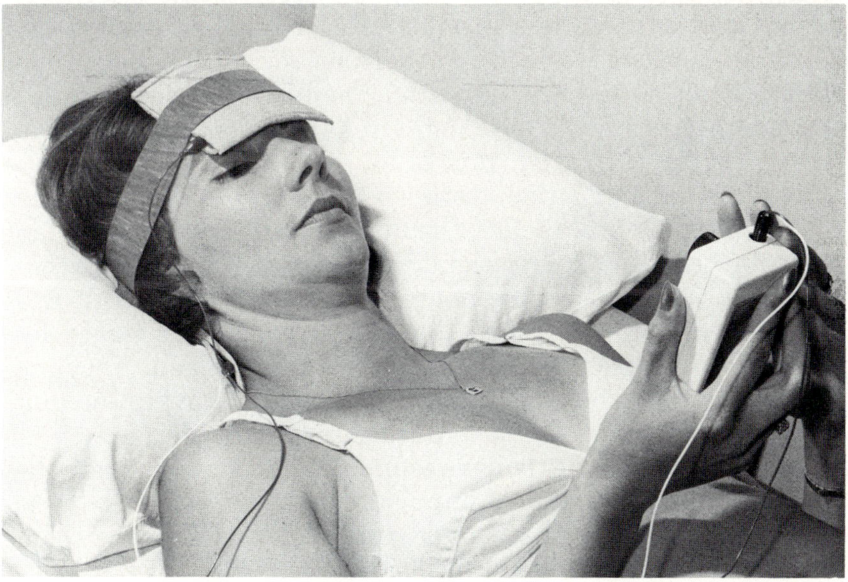

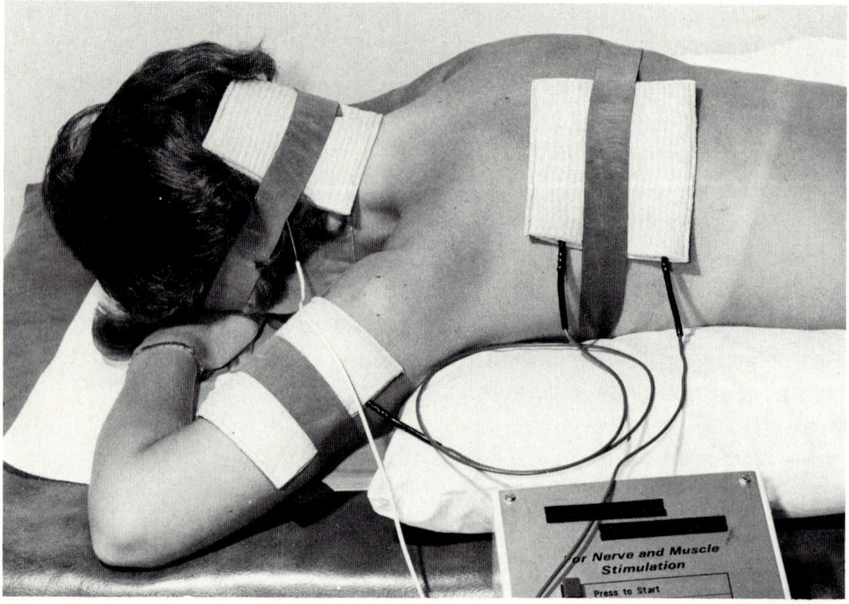

An initial attempt to reduplicate the referred pain pattern is advantageous in determining the potential effectiveness of the technique and frequently when the pain pattern can be reduplicated completely traumatic relief can be afforded.

The patient, once familiar with the application of the electrode, can usually determine the most effective site whether it be proximal or distal to a specific "trigger zone" of tenderness.

If the patient receives no benefit on the initial application after a period of several hours trial, the testing is discontinued and another series of "trial and error" sites can be chosen on succeeding days. If, after three or four days trial, no relief is afforded, further application testing does not appear appropriate.

If patients obtain relief, the unit was allowed to remain in place for between six and eight hours per day, usually discontinued during the sleeping hours. Occasionally, a patient will find it necessary to utilize the unit in the early stages for relatively prolonged periods of time including sleep. They are not usually disturbed by the inconvenience of having the unit wires and electrodes in place during these periods.

Many times patients have found that they can tolerate the application of the electrical impulses during the working day so that they can reach a plateau of pain relief and allowing them to continue a productive work load capacity.

Pain relief, once the impulses have been discontinued, is extremely variable and at times 8-10 hours of relief occur and allow the patient to sleep comfortably without the incumbencing device. Others, however, may experience 1-2 hours of relief and find it necessary to reapply the unit at intervals during the day.

The patients become familiar with the technical problems that may arise in respect to "battery failure", broken lead wires, and the loss of effective interphase between the electrodes and skin.

Occasionally, areas of erythema, itching, and increased pain may occur at the site of prolonged electrode application. Usually, these reactions disappear quickly when the application site is changed and a steroid ointment applied to the involved area.

Care should be taken in cervical area applications that the electrodes not be placed near the carotid sinuses.

Many transcutaneous units are available each having specific wave patterns and each may have an undesirable sensation for a specific patient. It may be necessary to change units in order to affect an ideal combination suitable for a specific patient.

Occasionally, patients who have obtained relief from the use of a specific unit may over a period of time develop diminishing relief from application but by again changing units, relief may frequently be obtained by using a differing technique.

Although the patients become "addicted" to their unit, after prolonged use, it has been found that they can be weaned relatively easily and still maintain their activity and work load program effectively.

After relatively prolonged periods of use, anesthesia has been reported in areas to which the electrodes have been applied, but these are usually not disconcerting to the patient and over a period of time normal sensation appears to return. Many of the patients who have received an effective period of relief from the transcutaneous electrical impulse application have failed to receive similar relief from acupuncture programs and it is difficult to explain these variations as the probable mechanism of relief is similar in each of these techniques.

EXPERIENCE WITH CHRONIC PAIN SITUATIONS

One of the most common potential applications of the use of electrical impulses is to the patient experiencing chronic low back pain.

In one study, 90 patients were evaluated in respect to their response to electrical impulses, 50 using the technique on an ambulatory outpatient basis and 40 on an ambulatory in-patient "pain ward" setting.

Although there did not appear to be significant correlation between the duration of symptoms and the success of the program, several patients in whom pain existed for over 15 years prior to the application of the electrical impulses did not experience significant relief.

In an attempt to evaluate a patient's improvement, the use of subjective response to the program was used in determining specific group designation.

A patient would be asked to determine improvement in one of three categories: 1) medication; 2) tolerance to activity and/or; 3) ability to work.

An excellent result was considered if a patient showed improvement in all aspects, a good result if he improved in two and only fair if improvement was present in a single category.

Almost half of the patients in the low back category had signs and symptoms suggesting some degree of residual nerve root irritation. Most patients, despite what apparently were adequate bony fusions at the desired level, appear to have symptoms due to mechanical strain patterns that were "stress aggravated and rest relieved".

The effectiveness of the unit would vary in respect to sites chosen for initial application of the electrodes. Most patients appear to derive maximum benefit with the application in the lower lumbar area but in those in which sciatic radiating pain was significant peripheral application to the posterior buttock or thigh area might be necessary to afford complete relief. The use of vertical electrodes covering several lumbar segments was also effective in several cases in blocking segmental rootlet pain.

Reference to (Table 1) appears to indicate that good and excellent results appear to have been obtained in patients under "ward" settings possibly because these patients received more intensive application of the unit, more thorough indoctrination as to the sites and methods of electrode application.

In respect to cervical syndrome problems, again approximately 40% appear to be relieved of their symptoms while undergoing inpatient indoctrination programs (Table 2).

Comparing the application of the electrical impulses technique to those patients experiencing both neck discomfort as well as headache (Table 3), there was no significant change in the end result percentages of the patients classified good and excellent. The use of the electrical impulses program for the relatively subcutaneous joints of knees and wrists appeared to afford some relief in arthritic conditions and certainly to the extent of considering these techniques for further application and study. (Table 4)

The application in post-herpetic neuralgia had been disappointing but the more recent literature is much more encouraging when patients with these conditions use TENS as a much earlier state in their disease process (Table 6).

Phantom pain and causalgic-like syndromes have been extremely difficult to counteract on a non-invasive basis and their responses to TENS have been encouraging even though variable (Table 5). It appears that more constant use of the unit in causalgic and phantom pain syndromes is warranted in view of the persistent pain patterns that have developed possibly within sympathetic chains.

TABLE 1
LOW BACK SYNDROME

	Inpatient	*Outpatient*
Unimproved	20	30
Fair	0	5
Good	12	8
Excellent	8	7
Total	40	50

TABLE 2
CERVICAL SYNDROME

	Inpatient	*Outpatient*
Unimproved	10	4
Fair	2	1
Good	4	5
Excellent	4	1
Total	20	11

TABLE 3
NECK AND HEADACHE—32 PATIENTS

	Inpatient	*Outpatient*
Unimproved	4	10
Fair	0	4
Good	5	5
Excellent	1	3
Total	10	22

TABLE 4
ARTHRITIS—RHEUMATOID AND OSTEOARTHRITIS
OUT-PATIENT THERAPY

	Knees	*Wrist*
Unimproved	1	1
Fair	1	1
Good	2	1
Excellent	1	0
Total	5	3

TABLE 5
PHANTOM PAIN—SIX PATIENTS
OUTPATIENT THERAPY

Unimproved	2
Fair	1
Good	1
Excellent	2

TABLE 6
POST HERPETIC NEURALGIA—FOUR PATIENTS
OUT-PATIENT THERAPY

Unimproved	2
Fair	1
Good	1
Excellent	0

CONCLUSIONS

The use of the transcutaneous electrical neuro stimulation technique is attractive for clinical application because of its dramatic and many times, complete relief of pain in situations where the more conventional methods have failed.

After appropriate training, the program is self-administered, self-supervised, and frequently gradually discontinued at the patient's discretion.

It is basically free of complications with the exception of temporary skin irritations that respond to discontinuing or alternating the sites of application.

Although addicted because of its effectiveness in the early stages, a patient can be weaned gradually from its application and frequently experience minimal, if any, return of pain.

Photos supplied by Bio Electronics Manufacturing Company.

Chapter 17

A DESCRIPTIVE SURVEY OF AVAILABLE T.E.N.S. DEVICES

GAIL H. BAUMGARTNER, A.B.

While reading the text and editing the contributions to this book, I became keenly aware of the cross-section of pain patients aided by T.E.N.S. and believed that an open listing of the varied types of instruments on the market today would prove beneficial to the pain patient and physician.

Twenty-seven manufacturers of T.E.N.S. devices were contacted and sent a one-page questionnaire relative to the products they currently market. Eighteen responded. Some supplied us with far more material than requested. Saul Liss, of the Pain Suppressions Labs, Inc., forwarded copies of papers presented at the Conference on Pain Management, Des Plaines, Illinois, May 14 & 15, 1977. This meeting was sponsored by the Pain and Health Research Institute and American Society of Contemporary Medicine and Surgery - Chicago, and St. Francis Hospital, LaCrosse, Wisconsin. Mr. William J. Lamers, Dip. A.P.A., Dip. V.M.P., Member of the Victorian Society of Medical and Biological Engineering, Victoria, Australia, discussed the usages of T.E.N.S. in the care of sporting and pet animals. They use it on greyhounds, for example, prior to races, with great success. Part of the information from Lamers was in the form of a tape.

Dan-Sjö Elektronik, of Sweden, and the Electronic Research Devices Corporation, Portland, Oregon, Bio-Electronics Manufacturing Company, Australia, Pain Suppression Labs of New Jersey and Med General of Minneapolis, MN supplied us with charts and photographs which are incorporated into the text. Mr. Dave Stanton, Medtronic, Minneapolis, MN. provided me with his latest paper (6/13/77) on the "Rationale for Constant Current Output" considering skin impedance and the skin's inherent complex electrical characteristics.

In mentioning the above cited individuals and companies, we are not endorsing one company over another. Instead, I want to thank them for supplying the langiappe which may be of benefit to many in the future.

The companies responding, and a summary of the response follows; they are listed alphabetically.

1. Avery Laboratories, Inc.
   Address: 145 Rome Street
   Farmingdale, New York 11735
   Telephone: 516-293-3630
   Trade names of Avery devices: *Avery T.E.N.S. system*
   Features: 2 & 4 leads, variable pulse width, amplitude and rate. Their unit has an alternating bi-directional square wave. Peak current is 30 milliamperes. Power source - rechargeable Nicad Batteries, with a charge life of from four hours at maximum setting to several days. Dimensions - 3 cm x 3 cm x 13 cm. Weight, 11 oz including battery pack.

2. Bio-Electronics Manufacturing Company
   Address: 109 Buckley Street, Essendon 3040, Australia
   Telephone Number: 370 6729
   Trade names of Bio-Electronics devices: *Bio-Stim & Painblok*
   Features: Two leads, with variable pulse width, amplitude and rate, with an adjustable rhythmical amplitude cycle; square wave form. On their professional model (11BM) stimulator which is designed for several usages, 1) Nerve Impulse Stimulation- uses low voltage direct current of single pulsed square wave potentials. 2) Acupoint Stimulation - low voltage alternating current of single spiked square wave potentials. 3) Spinal Segment Stimulation -

uses a low voltage alternating current of multiple pulsed square wave potentials.

They use both disposable and rechargeable batteries. The weight of the personal model is .375 kg and size 3 cm x 6 cm x 10.5 cm. Professional model weighs 4 kg. Dimensions 36 cm x 10 cm x 20 cm.

This company manufactures a number of devices, and develops others according to individual specifications. In addition to pain alleviation in humans, they have found it most useful in treatment of racing greyhounds and horses prior to races, post trauma, and in wound and bone healing in animals. On their in-clinic models, a shield may be used to block out the "hash" or stray noise from micro-, short, and long wave interferences. (Lamers - personal communication.)

3. Dan-Sjö Elektronik AB
   Address: Box 144
   S-172-24 Sundbyberg 1 Sweden
   Telephone: 08-98-32-60
   Trade names of Dan-Sjö Elektronik AB Devices: *Neurostal TNS* and *Travisens TNS Stimulator* 2 channels.
   Features: One model with two, one with four leads; one with, one without variable pulse width; both have variable amplitude and rate; square wave form; DC current max. 45 mA; power source is 9 volt rechargeable battery or accumulator. The life of charge is 2-3 weeks. Size - 59 x 29 - 104 mm. Weight - 170 g including battery. These dimensions are for the personal model.

4. Eigen Systems, Inc.
   Address: P.O. Box 1027, Grass Valley, CA 95945
   Telephone: 916-273-0067
   Trade Name of Device manufactured by Eigen: *Alpha III*
   Features: Two leads, amplitude 0-45 mA, rate 30-200 pulses/sec, pulsed wave form with a 9 volt alkaline battery as the power source. This is not rechargeable. The dimensions of the Eigen device are 14 x 5 x 2 cm. Weight, 120 grams.

5. Electronic Research Devices Corporation
   Address: 7380 SW 40th Avenue
   Portland, Oregon 97219
   Telephone: 503-245-2694
   Trade Name of Device Manufactured by Electronic Research devices: "*Load Sentinel*;; Transcutaneous Nerve Stimulating System
   Features: 2 leads (4 lead device available after July 1, 1977), variable amplitude (calibrated in MA, 0-30), rate fixed at 100 pps, and modulation with pulse bursts variable from .5 to 2 bursts per second. The wave form is square (bi-polar, symmetrical with constant current waveform). No DC current. The power source is 3 "A" Ni-Cad Rechargeable cells; the life of charge is 10-12 hours normally with MA control near 20. 6 hours with MA control at 30. There is a fast rate capability for re-charge; less than 6 hours for full recharge. The device is supplied with 6 batteries, removable for continuous operation at full intensity. The dimensions of the ERD Load Sentinel are 2⅞" x 4⅞" x ⅞", weighing 7 oz. with rechargeable batteries.
6. Elmed Incorporated
   Address: 60 West Fay Avenue
   Addison, Illinois 60101
   Telephone: 312-543-2792
   Trade Name of device distributed by Elmed:
   Intertronic Systems Ltd. (I.S.L.) *Neuroblock* cf.#8
   Features: Both two and four leads, variable pulse width, rate; wave shape-biphasic, spiked amplitude and;/D.C. Current, with a rechargeable battery pack, and charge life of 8 hours.
7. Frey Electronics, Inc.
   Address: P.O. Box 23391
   Tigard, Oregon 97223
   Telephone: 503-620=2722
   Trade Name of device manufactured by Frey:
   Bipulse Microstimulator - Model ST 1000 (formally nomenclated Neurex Bipulse Microstimulator.
   Features: 2 lead device, with fixed pulse width (at 75 microseconds), variable amplitude and rate. They believe the identical but opposite pulses eliminate the effects of electrolysis due to

positive ion build-up at one electrode and negative ion build-up at the other electrode. Waveform is described as pulsed or rectangular. Power source is 2 rechargeable nickel-cadmium cells; 2.5 v; recharge time approximately 8 hours, operating life up to 16 hrs.; dimensions- 2¼" x 2½" x ⅝". Their feeling is the very small size makes it more suitable to utilization of two separate units. (Mr. Harry Short of Med Dynamics, in San Francisco, California also responded with information on the Bipulse Microstimulator. He is connected with a manufacturing firm selling the device.)

8. General Medical Industries
   Address: 969 Barcelona Drive
   Santa Barbara, California 93105
   Telephone: 805-687-0483
   Trade Name of devices manufactured by General Medical Industries: GI-1212-1, GI-1212-2, GI-1212-3 (Little Black Box), GI-1212-6, GI-1007-1, GI-1007-2, and GI-1007-3
   Features: GI-1212-1, GI-1212-2, and GI-1212-3 each have one pair of leads. GI-1212-1 and GI-1212-2 have full frequency, while GI-1212-3 has variable pulse width and amplitude. GI-1212-6 has 4 leads, biphasic wave form, adjustable frequency. Dimensions on these are 2" x 2" x 1"; wt. 3½ oz. GI-1007-1 is a battery operated neurological stimulator used for sleep-research. Dimensions - 8" x 7" x 3"; wt. 3 lbs. (All of the 1212 series are battery operated as well.) GI-1007-2 has 3 pairs of leads, variable frequency, is battery operated; dimensions - 8" x 7" x 3"; wt. 3½ lbs. GI-1007-3 with 6 pairs of electrodes, rechargeable battery, timer, surge rate, switched frequency pulsation, biphasic wave form is used clinically after cosmetic surgery. They feel because of their electrode pads their skin problems are non-existent.

9. Intertronic Systems, Limited
   Address: 980 Alness Street, Unit 15
   Downsview, Ontario, M3J 2S2
   Telephone: 416-661-3902
   Name of devices manufactured by Intertronic: *Neuroblock*, *neuroprobe* cf # 6

Features: 2 & 4 lead devices with variable pulse width between 50 - 150 microseconds, amplitude 0-35 milliamps, 0-3500 ohms, rate 10-100 C.P.S., wave form - modified square wave, spiked; current - D.C., power source 4 AA cells, Nicad or Alkaline, life of charge 150-200 hours on 4 AA Alkaline at maximum output on both channels; optional rechargeable batteries; life of charge, 35-50 hours on 4 AA Nicad, 550 MAH capacity; size 2¾″ x 4½″ x 1″. No weight given.

10. Med General, Incorporated
Address: 10800 Lyndale Avenue South
Bloomington, MN 55420
Telephone: 612-888-8656 or 800-328-2847-toll free 24 hrs.
Names of Devices manufactured by Med General: *Microceptor, Miniceptor, Maxiceptor, Ceptor-Trodes* or *Post-op Electrodes*
Features: The Microceptor, with variable pulse width, amplitude and rate, square wave form, with Nickel-Cadmium and Alkaline rechargeable battery pack (micro-batteries with 15 hours of effective output at normal settings measures 2.65″ x 1.84″ x .65″ and weighs 2.3 oz. The Miniceptor I, with rectangular DC pulse shape and variable width, amplitude and rate, and rechargeable batteries, single channel, weighs 6.2 oz. with clip, measuring 1″ x 2″ x 4″.24 hr output. The Miniceptor II - dual channel stimulator has similar features but weighs .1 oz. more. 18 hr. output. Their largest model, the Maxiceptor, is a dual channel instrument permitting continuous or intermittent stimulation. It may also be used for muscular stimulation. It has a biphasic asymetrical square wave, adjustable pulse rate width, and amplitude, operating on a rechargeable 5 volt nickel-cadmium power pack. 20 hr. output. This device measures 5″ x 3″ x 15/16″, weighing 9.0 oz. Med General also produces the Ceptor-Trode, sterile, pregelled, self adhering T.E.N.S. electrodes for use in post-op control of pain. These electrodes which measure 2½″ x 7″ come with built in lead wires, ready for instant application.

11. Medical Devices, Inc.
    Address: 833 S.W. Third Street
    Saint Paul, Minnesota 55112
    Telephone: 800-328-0875- toll free, 612-631-0590
    Trade name of device manufactured by Medical Devices: *Neuropac I, Neuropac II, Neuropac III, Neuropac IV*
    Features: The Neuropac I, II, and IV have a non-symmetrical biphasic wave. I and II have adjustable amplitude and frequency; IV has adjustable pulse width as well. I, which has a single channel, weighs 8 oz; II and IV are dual channel, weighing 9 oz.

    III is a single channel device with adjustable amplitude, frequency and pulse width; this model's output waveform is a symmetrical biphasic squarewave. III weighs 6 oz. All models have rechargeable Ni-Cad batteries. Life of charge - 72 hours.
12. Medtronic, Inc.
    Address: 3055 Old Highway Eight
    Minneapolis, Minnesota 55418
    Telephone: 612-631-2860
    Trade names of TENS devices manufactured by Medtronic: *Neuromod 3701* single channel system, *Neuromod 3702* dual channel system, *Epiductive Tape Electrode System.*
    Features: 3701 single channel has 2 leads ("Y" cables available, with variable pulse width, amplitude and rate. Biphasic square wave form. Output is constant current from 100 to 1000 ohm impedance. The power source is 3 AA cells - alkaline or nicad; charger and battery packs are available. Dimensions 3.75′ x 2.75′ x .93′; weight 143 grams without batteries.

    3702 dual channel system has four leads, but can be operated as a single channel with two leads. The pulse width is not variable. Amplitude and rate are variable. The wave form is biphasic spike wave. The output is constant current from 100 to 1000 ohms. Its power source is 3 AA cells, either alkaline or nicad, and charger and battery packs are available. This unit is 4.4″ x 2.8″ x .95″ weighing 150 grams without batteries.

The Epi-Strip Tape Electrodes are designed to stimulate a 1″ x 6″ area.

13. Neuronics, Incorporated
    Address: 104 East Oak Street
    Chicago, Illinois 60611
    Telephone: 312-649-1400
    Trade Names and Features of the Neuronics device: This device is in production now. It has the capability of being both a constant current and a constant voltage stimulator. Approximate production date - November, 1977. It will have 4 leads, variable pulse width, amplitude and rate; square wave form, DC current. The power source is 2 9 volt batteries which are rechargeable. This handheld device will measure 2½″ x 4″ and weigh between 6-8 ounces.

14. N-Tron Electronics (formerly Neurotron Electronics)
    Address: 361 A Third Street, P.O. Box 3351
    San Rafael, California 94902
    Telephone 415-457-9060
    Trade names of devices manufactured by N-Tron: *Neurotron, N-Tron*
    Features: Two and four leads, with option to add additional piggypack leads. They have variable pulse width, amplitude and rate, with separate power controls for each channel giving the option to stack additional cables. The wave form is square, current A.C., power source 9 volt alkaline or 9 volt nickle cadmium rechargeable battery. This unit is approximately 3″ x 4″ x 1″, weighing 5¾ oz. with battery. Charge life 14 hrs/charge.

15. Owl Biomedical Incorporated
    Address: 901 Fuhrmann Blvd.
    Buffalo, New York 14203
    Telephone: 716-847-1340
    Trade name of device manufactured by Owl: *Delta C*
    Features: Two leads, variable amplitude and rate. The Delta C also comes with a plug in electrode to convert it to a hand held unit for stimulating larger areas. The wave form is trapezoidal. As a power source, it uses 4 mercury AA batteries, with the option of using rechargeable batteries. Dimensions are 13.0 cm x 6.4 cm x 2.8 cm.;

weight is 9 oz. Charge life 150 hours with mercury batteries.

16. Pain Suppression Labs, Inc.
    Address: 1200 Route 46
    Clifton, New Jersey 07013
    Telephone: 201-778-6000
    Trade names of devices manufactured by Pain Suppression Labs: Compact, portable *Pain Suppressor Model GL 105, Multi-person Multi-site Pain Suppressor Model GL 108*
    Features: Single knob control for variable intensity, this machine provides constant current, as set by the intensity control, over a range of skin resistance. The piggyback leads provide for stimulation of multiple sites. The power source is from 3 9 volt batteries, which last up to three months. Size - 3⅜″ x 3½″ x 5¾″. Weight - 20 oz. Battery life - 3 months.

    Model GL 108 is designed for professional use. This model has a single knob intensity control, adjustment timer, and rechargeable batteries lasting up to two years. Its output current provides constant current, as set by the intensity control, over a range of skin resistence. It may be applied to one or two persons simultaneously. Because of its design for clinical usage, it is larger than others. Size - 10¾″ x 14″ x 10″; weight approx. 20 pounds.

17. Staodynamics, Inc.
    Address: 601 South Bowen Street
    Longmont, Colorado 80501
    Telephone: 303-772-3631
    Trade Names of Staodynamics devices: Staodyn 2200, Staodyn 4400
    Features: 2 & 4 leads, variable pulse width, amplitude, rate; rectangular wave form. Current-zero net D.C. component to prevent iontophoresis. Power source 1 AA battery - rechargeable gives 20 hours; 1 AA battery - alkaline gives 100 hours. Dimensions - .69" x 1.92" x 2.35"; wt. 2.2 oz. They note that one of their patents (U.S. Patent 4,014,347) describes a unique combination of elements which provide maximum stimulation without electrical sensation.

18. Stimulation Technology, Inc.
Address: 9440 Science Center Drive
Minneapolis, Minnesota 55428
Telephone: 612-535-0255
Trade names of devices manufactured by Stim Tech: *EPC Mini, EPC Mini Dual, EPC Personal, EPC Personal Dual, EPC Clinical.*
Features: All Stim Tech EPC Stimulators have a modified rectangular pulse with zero net DC component. All have variable pulse width, amplitude and rate. The EPC Mini models have a rechargeable battery feature. This model takes 4 "AA" or "A" cells, and measure 1″ x 3″ x 5″, weight - 12 oz. The EPC Personal models use 3 "D" cell (flashlight batteries). This model measures 6″ x 5½″ x 2½″, weight 3 lbs. Battery life depends on parameters chosen.

The EPC Clinical Stimulator has the above features, but is dual channel, with an output disabler for a step on output of 15 ma or greater. The batteries are rechargeable. This device is designed for clinical use.

The above listings present an overall survey of the types of devices being marketed today. As Dr. Shealy points out in Chapter 5, several units may have to be tried for individual patients before the optimum one is selected.

It is evident from the differences in the described products that there is room for selection. But all have the common aim - increased comfort for the person with an acute or chronic pain problem.

Not all companies responded to the questionaire.
The following is a list of those companies:

Bio-Dyne Corporation, Chicago, Illinois 60611
Citronex, Walnut Creek, California 94596
Daltron, Mequon, Wisconsin 53092
Designs in Medicine, Mequon, Wisconsin 53092
Electreat, Incorporated, Minneapolis, Minnesota 55421
General Medical Industries, Santa Barbara, California 93105
Instrumentation and Control System, Incorporated, Addison, Illinois 60101
Neurostim Systems Limited, Scarbourough, Ontario M1R1K8

Nor Med, Seattle, Washington
J. A. Preston Corporation, New York, New York 10003

If any other companies have not been listed, it has been an oversight on our part. We checked and cross-checked our sources of information, and hope the data contained in this chapter will aid both physician and patient in their choice of instrumentation.

Most devices carry, either in their directions to the patient of physician, the disclaimer that use in pregnancy, with EEG, ECG or cardiac pacemakers is not established. The device is not to be emersed in water, or used without gel. Pulling off the electrodes without reducing dial settings may cause pain. If the electrodes remain in the same area for a prolonged period of time, a rash may develop, necessitating the change of gels or electrode sites.

Since these devices are to be prescribed only by a physician for treatment of one present pain syndrome, they should not be used, without the advice of a physician for other problems, or loaned to friends or neighbors. They are to be kept out of the reach of children, and used only as directed. When used in the proper manner, a significant number of pain patients will achieve the analgesia they seek.

Chapter 18

POST SURGICAL ANALGESIA WITH T.E.N.S.

JOSEPH G. BUSSEY, M.D., F.A.C.S.
AMY JACKSON, R.N., P.A.

Post surgical T.E.N.S. analgesia can supplement and frequently replace traditional pharmacological therapy. In an effort to determine its efficacy, we conducted a retrospective study of the modality, using 232 patients. Since 1974, we have been investigating and utilizing Transcutaneous Electrical Neuro Stimulation (TENS) permitting a post-surgical course with decreased pain. T.E.N.S. permits the patient to breathe deeply, cough, and increase his mobility. Narcotics slow down intestinal motility. The sedated patient's motion is decreased and respiratory effort impaired. With T.E.N.S. not only is analgesia achieved, but the complications of traditional pain therapy are reduced significantly.

We compared the amount of pain medication taken by consecutive patients on our service using the T.E.N.S. units with that taken by a control group. One hundred thirty-five patients had cholecystectomies, 75 inguinal hernioplasties, and 22 thyroidectomies. All procedures had been performed within the past 20 months at Atlanta West or Douglas General Hospitals, by board certified surgeons.

Specific pre-surgical patient training and hospital in-service education is directed by a full time nurse-technician. This staff member is skilled in demonstration and explanation of T.E.N.S. analgesic therapy. The nurse-technician also visits control patients, eliminating only that portion of pre- and post-operative instruction related to T.E.N.S.

Patients were eliminated who had known psychiatric or chronic pain problems, as were those being treated with T.E.N.S. pre-operatively for another pain state, or who were receiving opiates prior to surgery. Pregnant females and patients with demand type cardiac pacemakers were also excluded.

We found the results in this series statistically significant for the cholecystectomy and hernioplasty patients using the X^2 test, where $P < .001$. Using the appropriate Yates correction, a significantly higher proportion from the non-T.E.N.S. group required IM medication. However, the results in the thyroidectomy group are not of statistical significance at $P = .05$.

MATERIALS AND METHODS

The patients in this series ranged in age from 15 to 75. All individuals included were alert and oriented. Good results have been obtained with patients below the age of 15, but they were eliminated in an effort to concentrate on adult reactions to this modality. All patients were aware that pain medication (75 mg IM Demerol) had been ordered for them, should they need it following surgery.

The average age of the patients in the T.E.N.S. group who had cholecystectomies was 47 - 22 males, 28 females; average age in the control group - 45 - 37 males, 48 females. In the thyroidectomy patients, the control group age was 38 - 3 males, 7 females; the T.E.N.S. group 42 - 3 males, 9 females. The inguinal hernioplasty patients all were male. Average age of the control group was 40, of the T.E.N.S. group 42.

On the day prior to surgery, each patient in the T.E.N.S. group was visited by the nurse-technician on our team, trained in its usage. Introducing the patient to a brief background discussion of the concepts of electrical stimulation, she applied the electrodes from the T.E.N.S. unit to an area in close proximity to the proposed incisional site. In this series, we used the Microceptor T.E.N.S. units* (Fig. 1). This unit, measuring 2.65″ x 1.84″ x .65″ operates with a rechargeable battery pack as its power source, and provides the patient with the ability, by means of three dials, to regulate pulse width, rate and amplitude. Although the patients receive sufficient instruction to adjust their T.E.N.S. units completely, they rarely need to adjust the rate and width.

Once stimulation has taken place for several minutes, the patient is asked to pinch an area of skin between the electrodes, and report on the sensation experienced. Following performance of this "pinch test," when they do not experience pain from this site, they report on the sensation felt. In this way, the patient has a chance to experience the type of analgesia which he may expect post-surgically (1). The patient is also instructed to increase the dial settings until a sharp, painful stimulus is felt. In this way, he comes to know that this is the most unpleasant sensation he may expect from the unit, should the dials accidentally be turned incorrectly. Any questions the patient may have are discussed at this time, and he is instructed to contact the T.E.N.S. nurse should any arise. A notation is made on the pre-op work-up chart of the optimum dial settings. After experience with more than 1500 patients, we have determined the optimal setting to be Rate - 100 Hz (range 70 - 150 Hz); width - 100 msec. (range 60 - 150 msec); amplitude - quite variable but 80% of cases between 35 and 50 milliamps.

Following surgery, in the operating room, sterile electrode strips are placed several inches from the incision, with the electrodes placed closer to the spinal cord, if possible, in preference to a midline shift (Fig. 2). We seek to block several intercostal nerve segments, stopping pain not only from the incision, but from the contussed and bruised muscles which have been retracted. Additionally, we are striving to reduce the post-operative muscle spasms, an ongoing pain source. In dressing the area, elastic binders, which give compression support and secure the electrode strips, are used. When the patient reaches the recovery room, with the electrodes in place, the wires are attached to the T.E.N.S. unit, which is adjusted to the predetermined settings (Fig. 3).

The patient awakens in the recovery room with the unit attached and operating. Once he is transferred to his own room, he is visited daily by the T.E.N.S. nurse-technician, who checks on the function of the unit, re-explains, if necessary, the adjustment of the settings, should pain become perceptible, and answers any further questions. The rechargeable battery supplies are checked and the patient is told to call if there are any questions. Patients are encouraged to keep their units on continuously for the first 48 hours. After that, increasing periods without stimulation are recommended, thus using T.E.N.S. PRN, as one would with pain medication.

RESULTS

Patient acceptance of this modality has been enthusiastic. In comparing the amount of IM analgesic medication required by cholecystectomy patients with the control group, we find that on the day of surgery, the controls used 2.04 average doses of medication for pain versus 1.34 doses for the T.E.N.S. group; post-operative day #1 - 3.84 doses for the control group, 1.77 - T.E.N.S. group, post-operative day #2 - 3.18 controls, 1.29 T.E.N.S., post-operative day #3, 2.6 controls vs. 1.0 T.E.N.S. (Fig. 4). The hernioplasty patients in the control group on the day of surgery used an average of 1.74 doses vs. 1.33 for the T.E.N.S. group, an average of 2.35 injections for the controls versus 1.33 for the T.E.N.S. group on post-operative day #1, and 2.10 injections versus 1.0 on post-operative day #2. Control patients continued on post-operative day #3 to receive an average of 1.33 injections, while the T.E.N.S. group received none (Fig. 5). The control thyroidectomy patients used 2.14 average injections compared with 1.67 for the T.E.N.S. group, but the results are not statistically significant. (Fig. 6)

While limiting the comparison to IM analgesic medication, it is noteworthy that of the T.E.N.S. group, 3 patients requested and received 1 dosage each of p.o. Percodan for headache.

The pre-surgical discussion and preparation of the patient, who will use T.E.N.S., greatly enhances the outcome.

We also found it significant that in our T.E.N.S. group there were no complications of atelectasis or ileus. Since pulmonary embolization or ileus did not occur in any of the patients in the T.E.N.S. group, for accuracy in comparison, we eliminated from the control group any who had complications.

DISCUSSION

In 1965, Melzack and Wall proposed a theory of pain transmission which postulated that the fast conducting, large diameter fibers, when stimulated cause decreased perception of stimuli carried by slow conducting fibers. This was thought to occur via a gating mechanism in the substantia gelatinosa of the dorsal horns (2).

Sweet, Wall and Wepsic began the pioneer experimental investigations (3,4). Initially, it seemed that the most practical application of this theory lay in the area of chronic pain control. And indeed work was done first in the area of implanted dorsal column stimulators (5,6,7,8,9,10,11). When it became evident that a screening device to determine the potential efficacy of implanted stimulators was necessary, T.E.N.S. units first came into clinical usage. Patients, finding a significant degree of analgesia from chronic pain often opted to use the T.E.N.S. units rather than proceed with implantation. Thus, T.E.N.S. usage in the field of chronic pain grew.

In the past five years, several reports have appeared in the literature studying T.E.N.S. as a post-operative analgesic modality (12,13,14,15,16,17). Other studies in the European literature utilizing transcutaneous and percutaneous electrical stimulation have continued to support this form of therapy (18,19,20,21,22). It has also been noted that when T.E.N.S. is used in the treatment of protracted ileus, it may prove to be of value in differentiating between true ileus and mechanical obstruction (16).

We have examined T.E.N.S. for its relevance in the control and management of acute surgical pain. The trauma encountered in surgery is perceived via a direct electrical impulse transmitted via a nerve fiber, then through a synapse in the spinal cord, ascending through various tracts to the brain, where it is assimilated, and finally perceived by the cortex as pain.

If there is a stimulus which is sufficiently intense, repetitive, or of long duration, it can reset the mid-brain to perceive this input as continuing. T.E.N.S. usage can alter this process, alleviating acute discomfort and simultaneously minimizing the development of such chronic pain syndromes as post thoracotomy or phantom limb pain.

Selecting the patients for this series, we sought to compare T.E.N.S. utilization with the amount of standard post-operative analgesic IM medication. We found that the comparative differences were significant (Figs. 3-5).

An additional contributory factor to the success of our program has been the employment of a full-time nurse-technician, who instructs the patients pre- and post-operatively in the operation of the units, changing of batteries, and answers any questions which they may have regarding this type of therapy. She spends an average of 30 minutes with each pre-operative patient, and five to seven minutes on each post-operative day. Her instruction and on-call availability enhance the success of this operation.

The in-house nursing staff also feel more at ease with this non-pharmacological analgesic method if they have someone with whom they may consult should a problem occur.

The nurse-technician is also responsible for in-service education of the nursing staff of the hospital, and careful instruction of the recovery room nurses. It is in the recovery room nursing reports that we find our most satisfying initial reaction, since they note that since the inception of T.E.N.S. usage, they no longer have to worry about giving any IM post-operative medication while the patient is in recovery.

Questions regarding post-surgical electrode placement continue. From our experience in T.E.N.S. usage, we have become increasingly aware that the initial dermatome mapping is too rigid. We find it may be best to try to block several intercostal nerve segments, since there may be a two or three segment variation between people, leading to uncertainty regarding which nerve to block to relieve pain at a given site. We prefer placement of the strip electrodes several inches from the incision, with a shift toward the spinal cord rather than the midline wherever possible.

Since the patients in the operating room are generally not sufficiently reactive to experience pain, we find attachment of the T.E.N.S. unit to the electrodes in the recovery room entirely satisfactory. The patient then awakens with the unit on and functioning, and the recovery room nurses have been thoroughly instructed by the T.E.N.S. nurse-technician as to specific settings, operation of the units, and what to do if a problem arises.

We have found that the patient who is pre-operatively trained in the use of the unit attains more analgesia than someone who wakes up in the recovery room with the unit on, unaware of its function. One cannot disregard the placebo effect. Certainly, the well-prepared patient experiences a diminution of anxiety. But patient instruction is given to both T.E.N.S. and controls, and there still remains the marked difference in the amount of medication needed.

Few of our post-operative patients take T.E.N.S. units home, but one experience we have had with our inguinal hernioplasty patients who are now returning home on post-operative day #3, rather than day #4 or #5, is that once they are back home, they become aware of how much analgesia they were getting from the "little box" and comment that it was not until they returned home that they realized how much help T.E.N.S. had been to them, and what pain had been blocked out.

SUMMARY

We have formulated the following observations based on over 1500 general surgical cases treated since late 1973. The data presented in this paper, however, has been accumulated since 1 January 1978.

1. Electrode placement in direct proximity to the incision is not necessary. Placement several inches from the incision is preferable.
2. Proper patient education prior to surgery and the employment of a nurse-technician skilled in patient education and evaluation is of utmost importance.
3. Education of general nursing personnel is necessary. They must learn that every post-operative patient does not need medication in order to be comfortable and pain free.
4. Neuroaugmentation is always superior to neuroablation, since in the latter there is a loss of access to the system. Using opiates and sedatives for post-operative pain management is equivalent to acute neuroablation. In the acute patient, over-sedation decreases deep breathing, coughing and extremity exercises necessary to prevent such complications as depressed pulmonary function and phlebothrombosis. The patient's active participation in post-operative recovery can be maintained by

using transcutaneous electrical nerve stimulation as the primary modality for pain control.

Although a relatively new concept in the field of acute pain control, Transcutaneous Electrical Nerve Stimulation has significantly decreased the amount of pain medication needed by patients on our general surgical service, and provided these patients with analgesia minus pharmacologic complications. Its employment in a general surgical practice has proven to be of significant patient benefit.

BIBLIOGRAPHY

1. Picaza, J., Cannon, D., Hunter, S., Boyd, S., Guma, J., and Maurer, D.: Pain suppression by peripheral nerve stimulation, Part I: Observations with implanted devices. *Surg. Neurol., 4:* 115-126, July 1975.
2. Melzack, R., and Wall, P.: Pain mechanisms: A new theory. *Science, 150:* 971-3, 1965.
3. Wall, P., Sweet, W.: Temporary abolition of pain in man. *Science, 155:* 105, 1967.
4. Sweet, W., and Wepsic, J.: Stimulation of the posterior columns of the spinal cord for pain control: Indications, techniques, results. *Clin. Neurosurg.,* 789-810. Proceedings of Col. of Neuros. Honolulu, 1978, Williams & Wilkins, Baltimore 1974.
5. Kirsch, W.D., Lewis, J., and Simon, R.: Experiences with electrical stimulation devices for control of pain. *Med. Instrument, 9* (5) 217-20, Sept., Oct. 1975.
6. Krainick, J.J., and Thoden, U.: Methods of pain modulation by electrical stimulation. *Langenbacks Arch Chir., 342:* 75-81, 1976.
7. Nashold, B., and Friedman, H.: Dorsal stimulation for control of pain. Preliminary report on thirty patients. *J. Neurosurg., 35* (5) 590, 1972.
8. Shealy, C.N., Mortimer, J., and Hagfors, N.: Dorsal column electroanalgesia. *J. Neurosurg., 32:* 560, 1970.
9. Long, D.: New methods of pain relief. *Minn Med, 55:* 565, 1972.
10. Long, D.: Electrical stimulation for relief of pain from chronic nerve injury. *J. Neurosurg., 39:* 718-729, 1973.
11. Sweet, W.: Specific Neurol Stimulation for inhibition of pain. *Pros. Aust. Ass. Neurol., 5:* 459-461, 1968.
12. Hymes, A., Raab, D., Yonehiro, E., Nelson, D., and Printy, A.: Acute pain control by electrostimulation: a preliminary report. *Advances in Neurology,* Vol. 4, International Symposium on Pain, Raven Press, N.Y., 1974.
13. Hymes, A., Yonehiro, E., Raab, D., Nelson, D., and Printy, A.: Electrical surfact stimulation for treatment and prevention of ileus and atelectasis. *Surg. Forum, 26:* 222-4, 1975.
14. VanderArk, G., and McGrath, K.: Transcutaneous electrical stimulation in treatment of postoperative pain. *Am. J. Surg., 130:* 338-40, 1975.
15. Cooperman, A., Hall, B., Mikalacki, K., Hardy, R., and Sadar, E.: Use of transcutaneous electrical stimulation in the control of postoperative pain: Results of a prospective, randomized, controlled study. *Am. J. Surg., 133:* 185-7, Feb. 1975.
16. Perdikis, P.: Transcutaneous nerve stimulation in the treatment of protracted ileus. *S. Afr. J. of Surg., 15:* (2) 81-6, June 1977.
17. Pike, P.: Transcutaneous electrical stimulation: Its use in the management of

postoperative pain. *Anaesthesia, 33:* 165-71, 1978.
18. Kurzbauer, R., and Kurzbauer, E.: Postoperative pain. *Pielgi Polozna* (9) 5-7, 1978.
19. Proshina, I.V.: Evaluation of use of the elektroson apparatus for postoperative analgesia. *Med Tekh,* (2) 53-3, Mar.-Apr. 1974.
20. Rasstrigin, N.M.: Electroanalgesia during the postoperative period in gynecological patients. *Med Sestra, 35* (11) 21-4 Nov. 1976.
21. Heftman, W.R.: Electrosleep and its use in surgery. *Pol Przegl Chir. 43* (7) 1185-91, Jul. 1971.
22. Mkrtichian, S.M.: Effect of electrosleep on the motility of the gastrointestinal tract. *Zh Eksp Klin Med., 15* (1) 84-8, 1975.

Chapter 19

CONCLUSION

ROBERT A. ERSEK, M.D.

Wall and Melzack's exploration into the concept of pain transmission led directly to studies conducted in a number of controlled situations. From the ideas substantiated by the Gate Control Theory, scientists began experimenting with implanted dorsal column devices. Percutaneous stimulation was tried, with some success. But the most significant work has been in the area of Transcutaneous Electrical Neuro Stimulation. This is a comfortable form of analgesia. There are few significant risks.

The pioneer work done by Sweet and Wepsic, Long, Shealy and others throughout the world gave us insights into this therapeutic device, testing this modality in controlled studies. Their favorable results led to its usage in the treatment of patients with acute and chronic pain.

Many of the patients are initially treated in pain centers. But it is also being used more frequently in sports related injuries. It was approved for use at the Olympic Games in Montreal in 1976. Large companies employ it in their physical therapy departments or clinics for analgesia in on the spot job-related injuries. Contemporary dentistry has seen its adaptability to specific pain problems. (Figure 1). It is adaptable for use in virtually every medical specialty, for clinic use, and in emergency departments.

Pain indicates pathology and its characteristics and location give us necessary data relative to its etiology and the proper course of treatment. Once the nature of the presenting pain syndrome is identified, and underlying pathologies considered, T.E.N.S. can supply as a fortuitous result, the cessation or diminution of suffering. Those patients who achieve

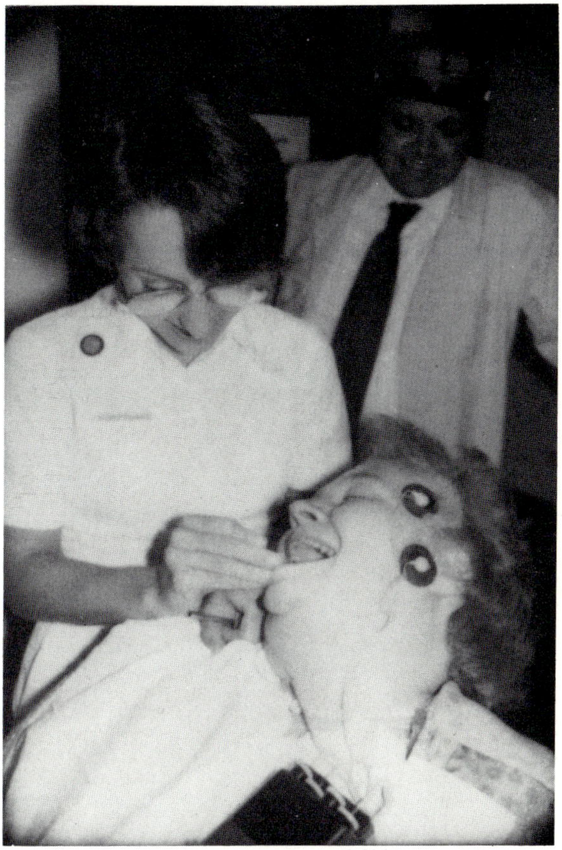

Figure 1
This illustrates the efficacy of T.E.N.S. in controlling pain in a dental procedure. Prior to utilization of T.E.N.S. during routine dental examination and cleaning, the patient suffered severe headaches, often lasting more than three days.

relief from this therapy will benefit most from continued research in this new, rapidly broadening field.

Our contributors to this book practice in a variety of specialty areas. But the experience of their direct studies and contact with T.E.N.S. have caused them to appreciate its worth, and to pool their knowledge and enthusiasm in the rapidly developing field of dolorology.

AUTHORS LIST

INDEX